COLOR ATLAS OF HUMAN ANATOMY

人体解剖彩色图谱

主编　扈燕来　孙晋浩　李贵宝

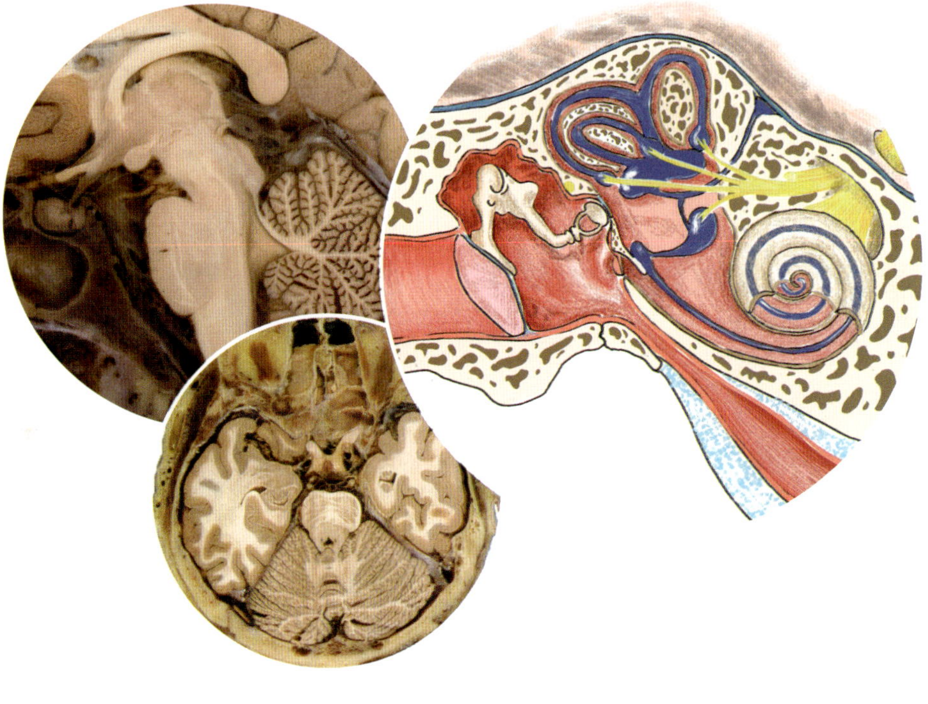

山东科学技术出版社

·济南·

图书在版编目（CIP）数据

人体解剖彩色图谱 / 扈燕来，孙晋浩，李贵宝主编. 济南 : 山东科学技术出版社，2025. 8. -- ISBN 978-7-5723-2609-7

Ⅰ. R322-64

中国国家版本馆 CIP 数据核字第 20254BG607 号

人体解剖彩色图谱

RENTI JIEPOU CAISE TUPU

责任编辑：李志坚
装帧设计：孙小杰

主管单位：山东出版传媒股份有限公司
出 版 者：山东科学技术出版社
地址：济南市市中区舜耕路 517 号
邮编：250003　电话：（0531）82098088
网址：www.lkj.com.cn
电子邮件：sdkj@sdcbcm.com
发 行 者：山东科学技术出版社
地址：济南市市中区舜耕路 517 号
邮编：250003　电话：（0531）82098067
印 刷 者：日照蓝图仕印务有限公司
地址：山东省日照市莒县招贤镇罗庄二路西路 3 号
邮编：276500　电话：（0633）7770369

规格： 16 开（184 mm × 260 mm）
印张： 21.75　**字数：** 409 千
版次： 2025 年 8 月第 1 版　**印次：** 2025 年 8 月第 1 次印刷
定价： 98.00 元

主　　编　扈燕来　山东大学齐鲁医学院
孙晋浩　山东大学齐鲁医学院
李贵宝　山东大学齐鲁医学院

副 主 编　徐广琪　山东省公共卫生临床中心
李志宇　山东第一医科大学附属省立医院
张　建　山东大学齐鲁医院德州医院
吴国君　山东第一医科大学附属省立医院
仇申强　山东第一医科大学附属省立医院
张建水　西安交通大学
张　萍　山东大学第二医院
陈　丹　山东中医药大学
宗　维　山东第一医科大学附属省立医院

编　　委　于云海　山东大学第二医院
王志勇　新乡医学院
王晓露　内蒙古医科大学
田广平　山东大学齐鲁医学院
史风雷　山东大学齐鲁第三医院
付廷刚　齐鲁医药学院
巩念明　山东第一医科大学
朱明昇　潍坊市人民医院
刘　真　山东大学齐鲁医学院
刘小菊　山东中医药大学
刘洪武　山东第一医科大学附属省立医院
刘晓光　湖南交通工程学院
刘稳柱　菏泽医学专科学校

汤煜春　山东大学齐鲁医学院
张　静　山东大学齐鲁医学院
汪　澎　山东大学齐鲁医院
孙丰刚　山东第一医科大学
吴龙祥　南昌医学院
宋天罡　山东大学第二临床学院
张　鑫　山东第一医科大学附属省立医院
陈　超　山东第一医科大学附属省立医院
陈京国　河北医科大学第三医院
殷　威　山东大学齐鲁医学院
殷庆丰　山东大学第二医院
韩　笑　南通大学
韩义成　山东第一医科大学附属省立医院
温明新　山东大学齐鲁医学院

标本制作人员　马广星　王　震　田广平　白　石　刘晓光　孙丰刚
李　鹏　李志宇　宋　涛　张俊峰　林兆恒　周启迪
相　皓　侯海光　秦成涛　徐海艇　高展鹏　郭中献
郭庆河　崔　斐

绘　　图　邢睿南　曹学飞　韩浩盈　闫姝睿　郑文琦　徐永杭
林国铭

摄　　影　邢长山　李贵宝　扈燕来

图片处理　邢长山　李佳艺　扈燕来

图片标注　于　漠　田　灿　吴梦璇　余睿萱　宋　瑞　宋天罡
张　敏　张奕祯　陈洪冰　胡莘悦　殷　威

前 言

人体解剖学是研究正常人体形态和构造的科学，既是重要的医学专业基础课程之一，又是联系基础医学与临床医学的桥梁课程。学好人体解剖学，对医学相关专业的学生来说，意义重大。一本图片详尽、清晰，标注准确、详细的人体解剖图谱，会使人体解剖学的学习事半功倍，将是医学相关专业学生的良师益友。

本书编写团队由国内多所院校和医院的解剖学教师和临床医生组成，严格按照统一标准收集各种实体解剖标本并摄制照片，紧密结合临床实际收集大量拓展阅读资料，安排专人进行中英文对照的详细标注，最终历时 4 年多完成了本书的编写工作。在此，对在本书编写工作中付出辛勤劳动的编写、制作团队表示衷心感谢。

本书内容紧扣临床医学专业五年制和“5+3”一体化规划教材的教学大纲和教学要求，分为系统解剖学和局部解剖学两个部分，前者按系统展示器官的形态结构，后者按部位展示局部解剖结构与层次，共收录包括实体解剖图片、解剖示意图等在内的彩色解剖图片近 600 幅，还可扫二维码获取相关电子资源。

本书的特色鲜明：①内容紧扣临床医学专业五年制和“5+3”一体化规划教材的教学大纲和教学要求，包括系统解剖学和局部解剖学；②扫描二维码，可获取电子影像资源，使人体解剖学知识与临床实际密切结合；③实体标本按照统一标准制作，解剖结构对比清晰，同时补充了其他图谱中欠缺的手、足、眼和脑干等的切面、灌注、染色图片，内容更加完善。

在本书编写过程中，刘树伟教授给予了大力支持并提供了宝贵的建议和意见；另外，部分医学院校的解剖学教师和医院的临床医生也提供了宝贵的指导意见和资料，在此一并表示衷心感谢。

由于时间仓促和经验有限，书中存在不当之处，敬请读者指出，我们会在修订、再版的过程中改正，对此表示衷心感谢。

编　者

第一章　运动系统

扫码获取电子资源

第一节　骨

第二节 骨连接

第三节 骨骼肌

第二章 消化系统

第三章 呼吸系统

第四章 泌尿生殖系统

第五章　心

第六章　淋巴系统

第七章 感觉器

第一节 视器

第二节　前庭蜗器

第八章 内分泌腺

第九章 神经系统

第十章 局部解剖

第十一章 头部、躯干和四肢断面

第一章　运动系统

第一节　骨

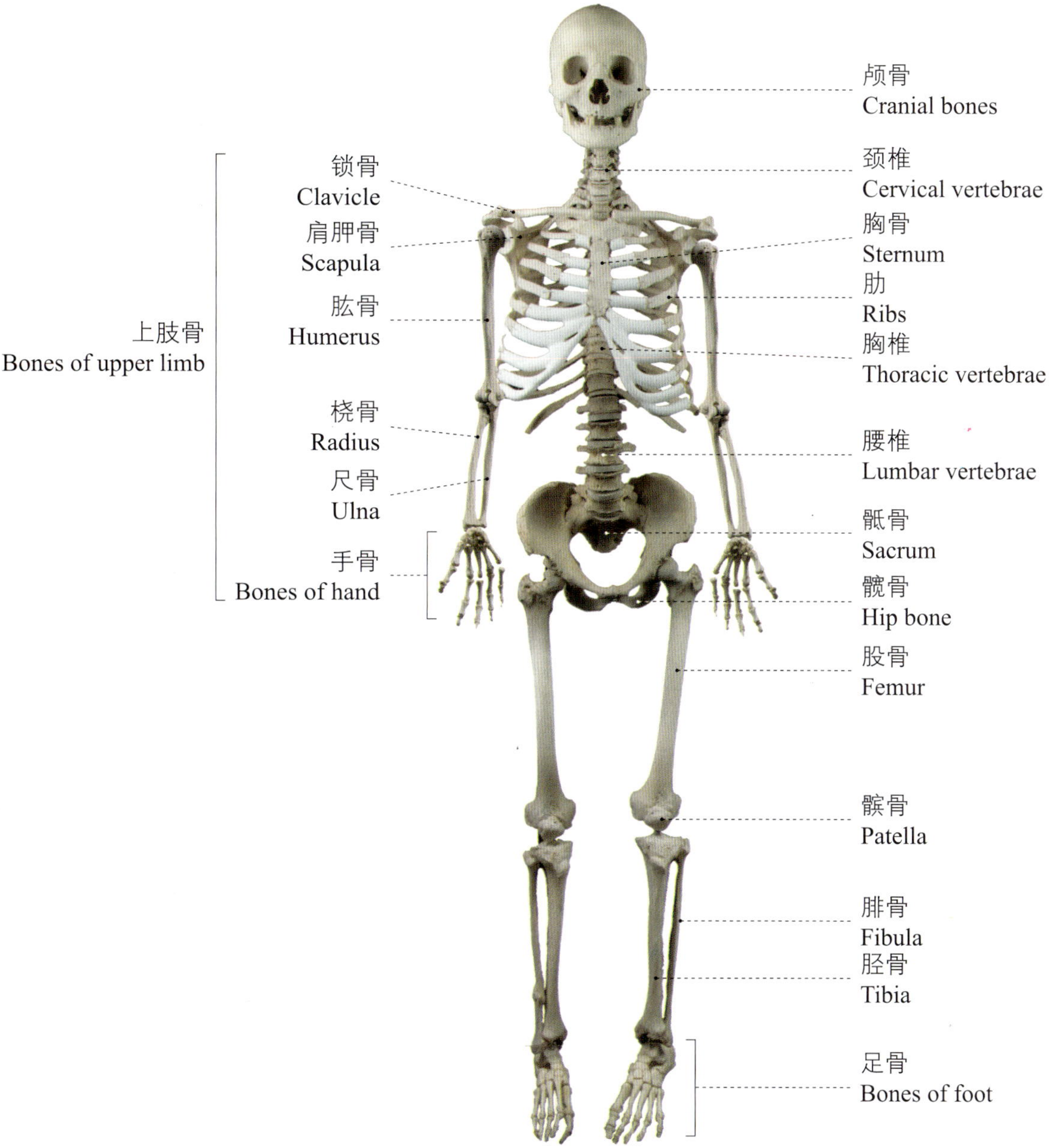

图 1-1　全身骨骼（前面观）

Skeleton. Anterior aspect

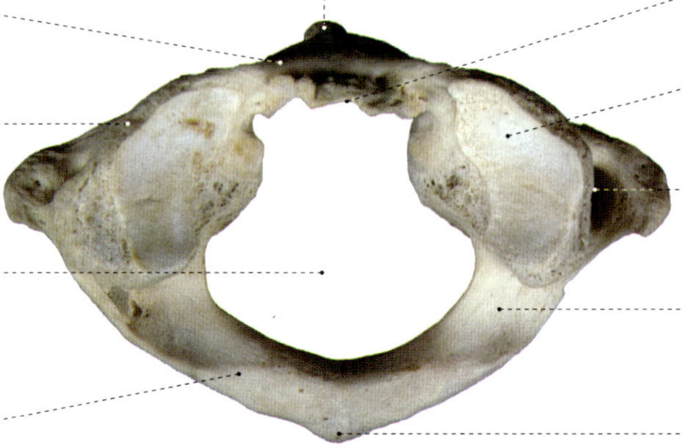

图 1–7　寰椎（上面观）

Atlas. Superior aspect

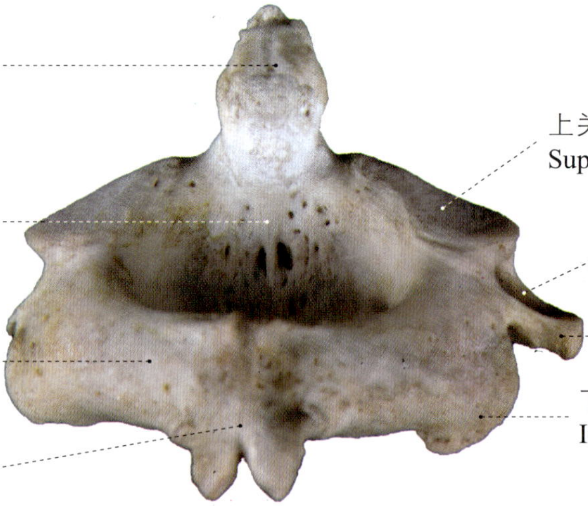

图 1–8　枢椎（后面观）

Axis. Posterior aspect

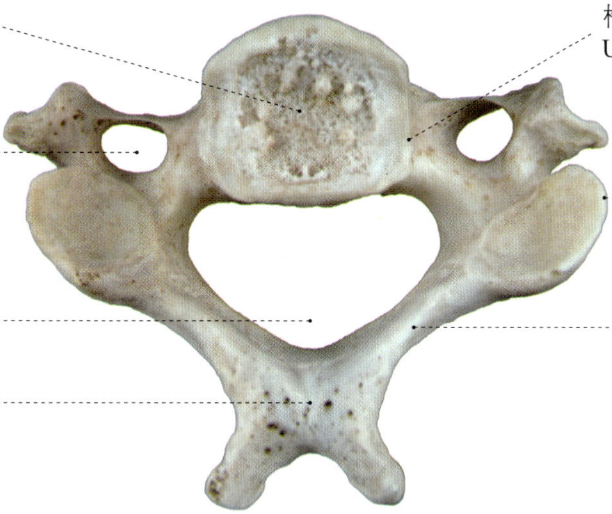

图 1–9 颈椎（上面观）

Cervical vertebra. Superior aspect

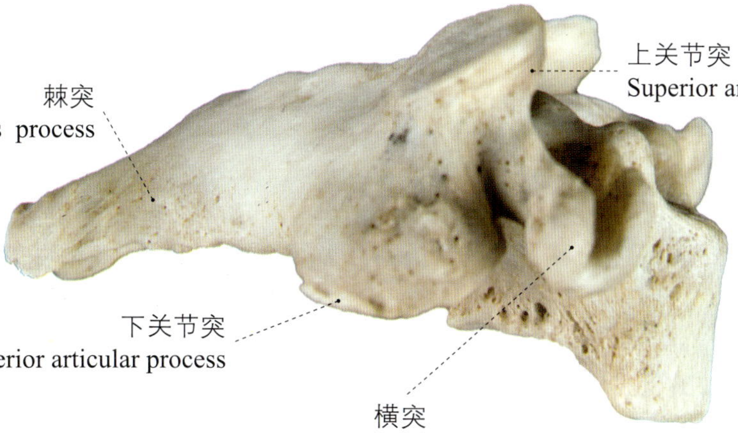

图 1–10 隆椎（外侧面观）

Vertebra prominens. Lateral aspect

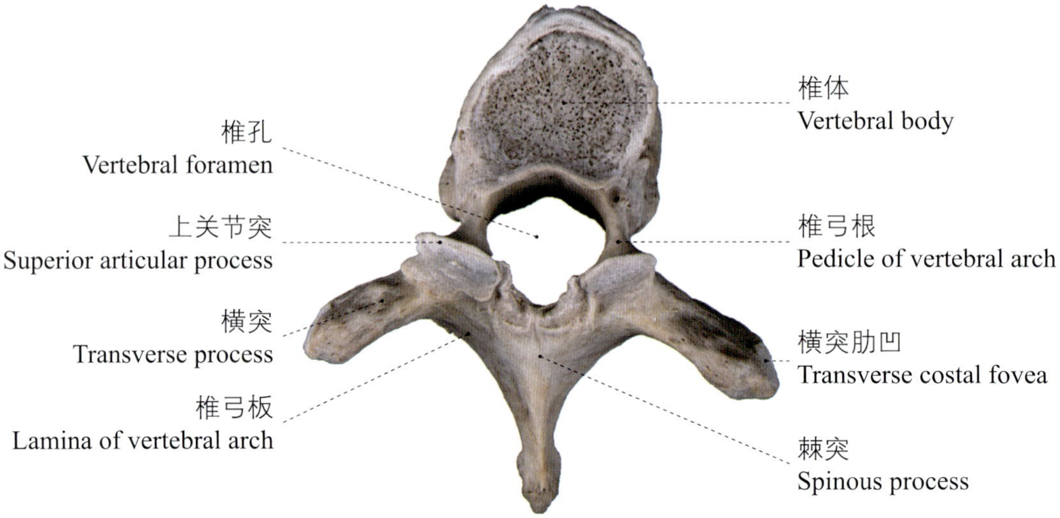

图 1–11　胸椎（上面观）

Thoracic vertebra. Superior aspect

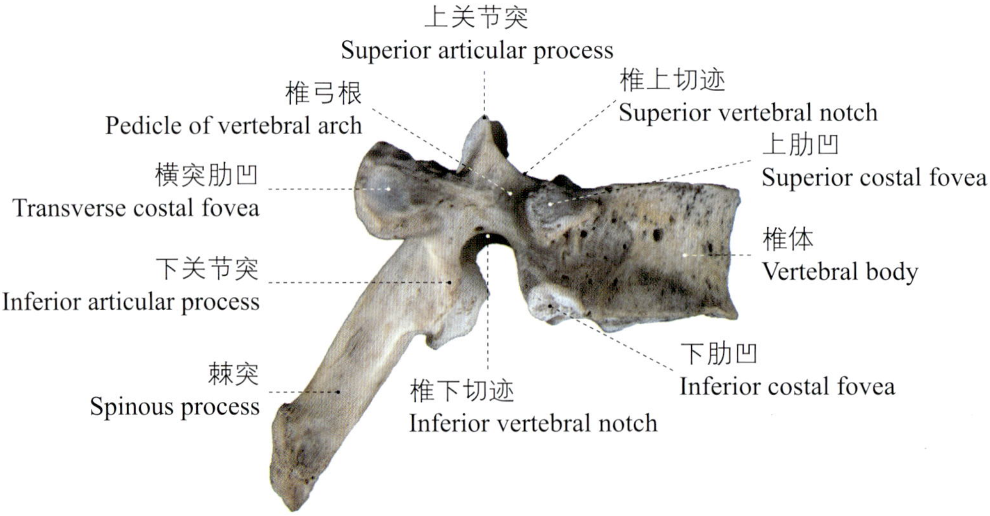

图 1–12　胸椎（外侧面观）

Thoracic vertebra. Lateral aspect

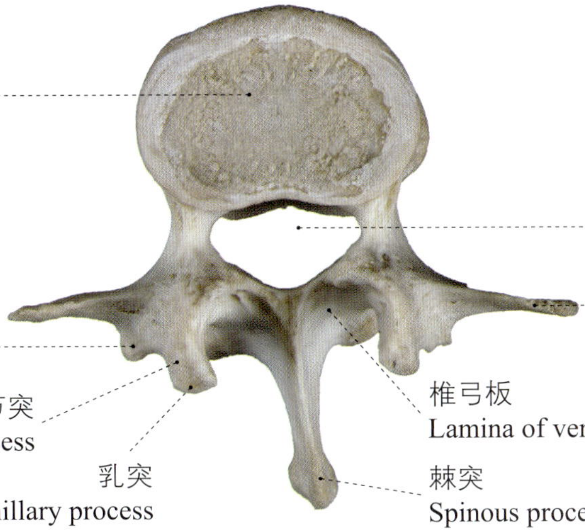

图 1–13　腰椎（上面观）

Lumar vertebra. Superior aspect

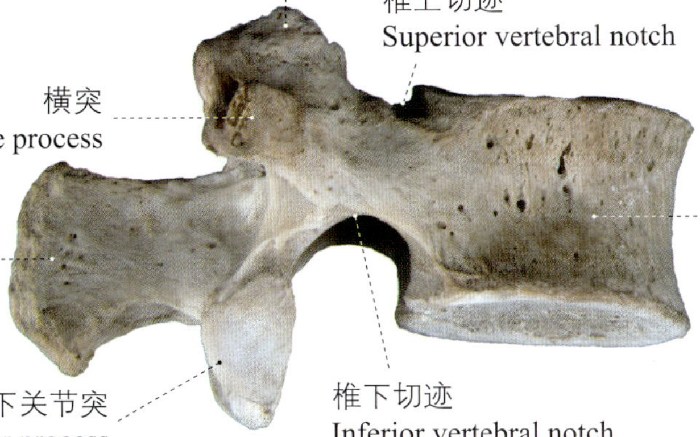

图 1–14　腰椎（外侧面观）

Lumar vertebra. Lateral aspect

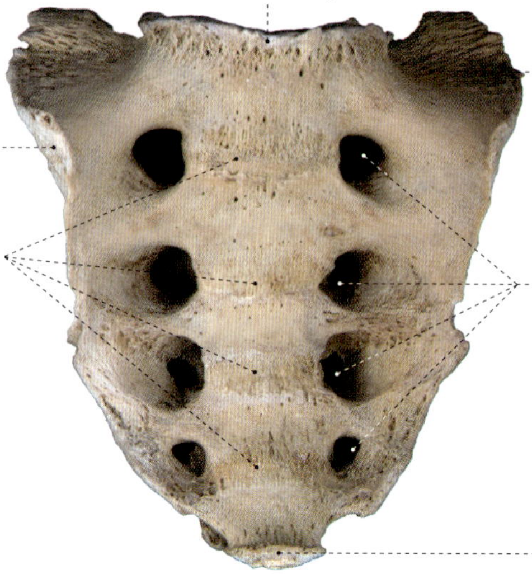

图 1–15 骶骨（前面观）

Sacrum. Anterior aspect

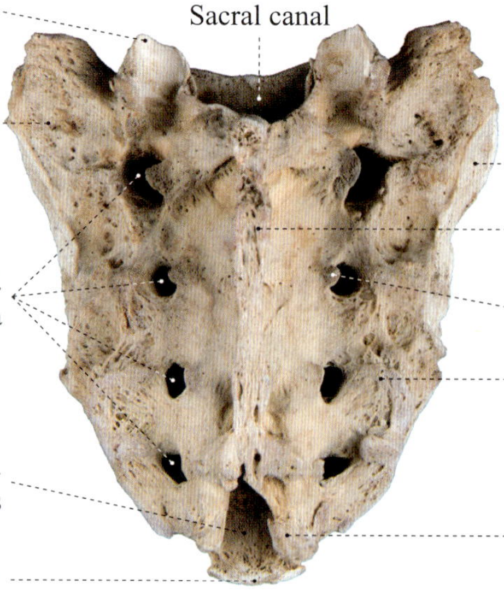

图 1–16 骶骨（后面观）

Sacrum. Posterior aspect

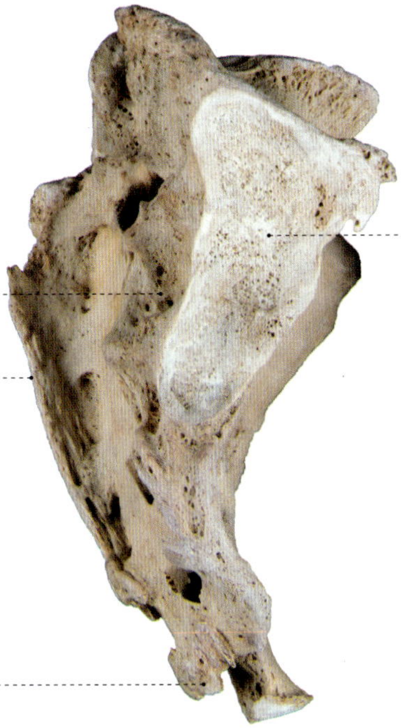

图 1-17　骶骨（外侧面观）

Sacrum. Lateral aspect

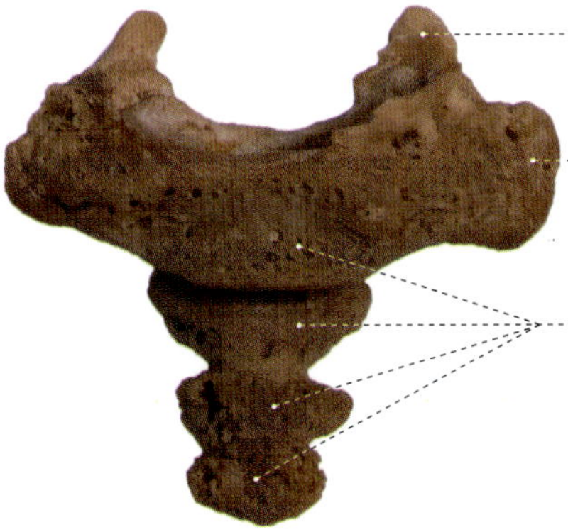

图 1-18　尾骨（前面观）

Coccyx. Anterior aspect

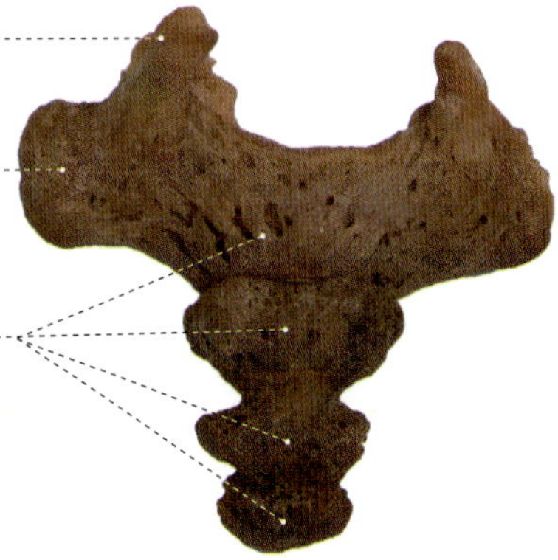

图 1-19　尾骨（后面观）

Coccyx. Posterior aspect

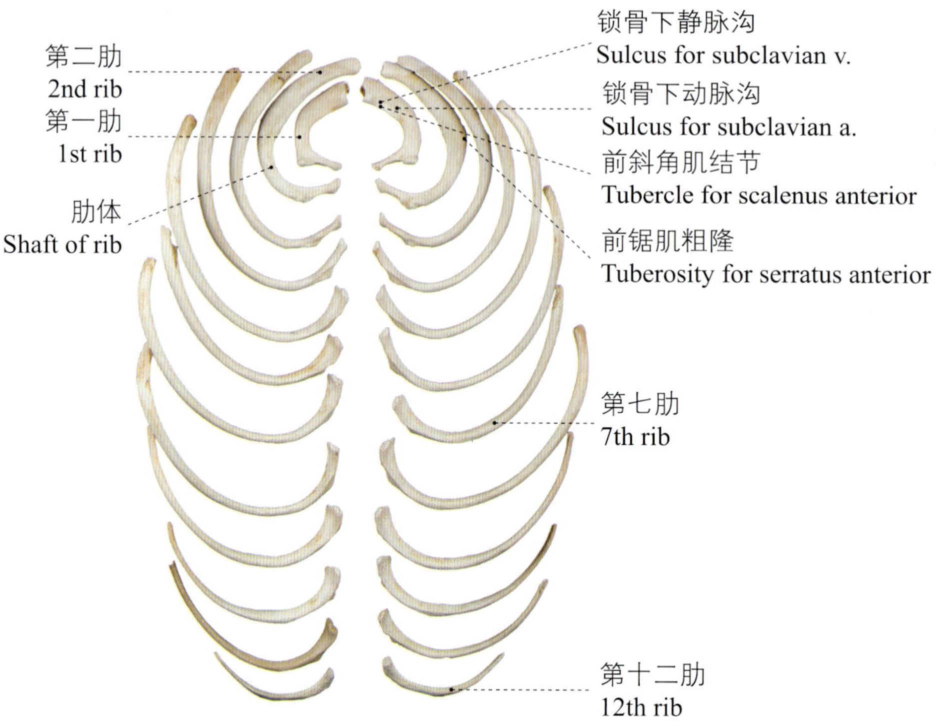

图 1–20　肋

Ribs

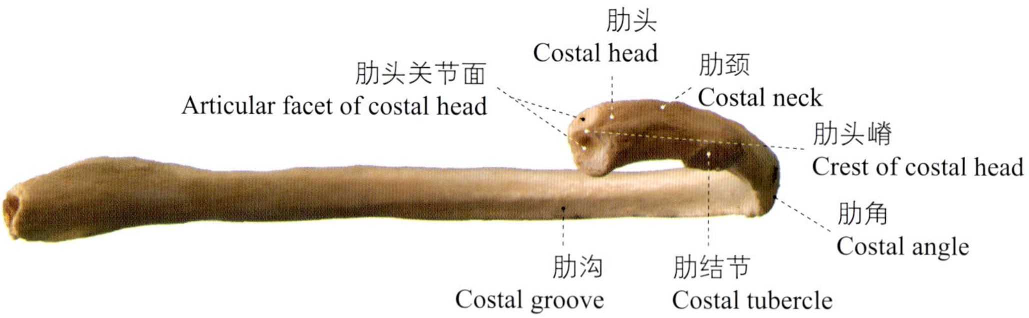

图 1–21　肋骨（内面观）

Costal bone. Internal aspect

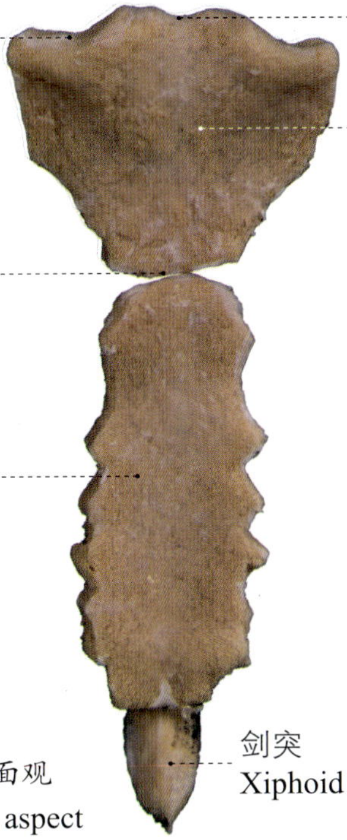

A. 前面观
Anterior aspect

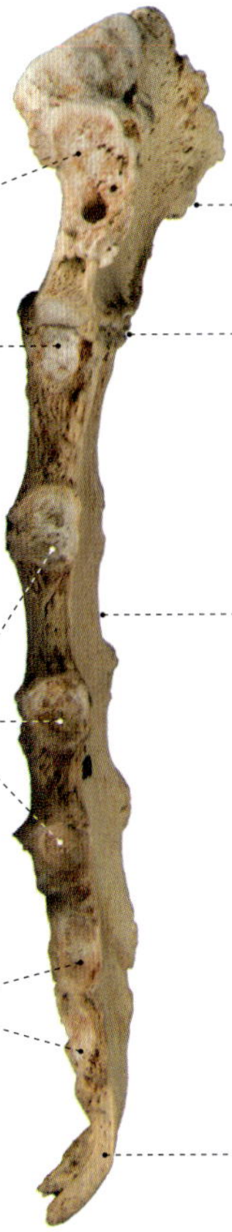

B. 外侧面观
Lateral aspect

图 1–22　胸骨

Sternum

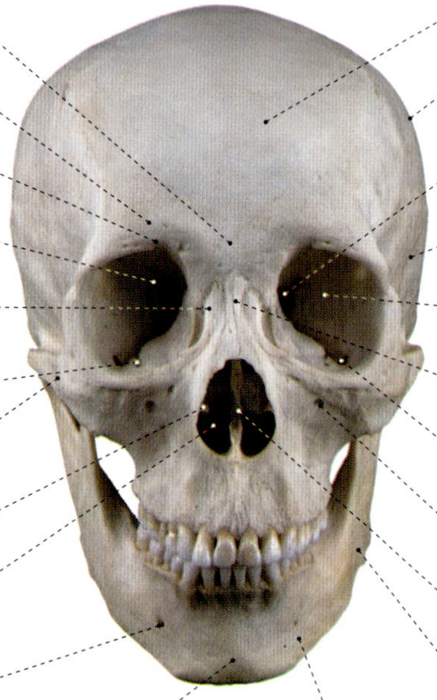

图 1–23　颅（前面观）

Skull. Anterior aspect

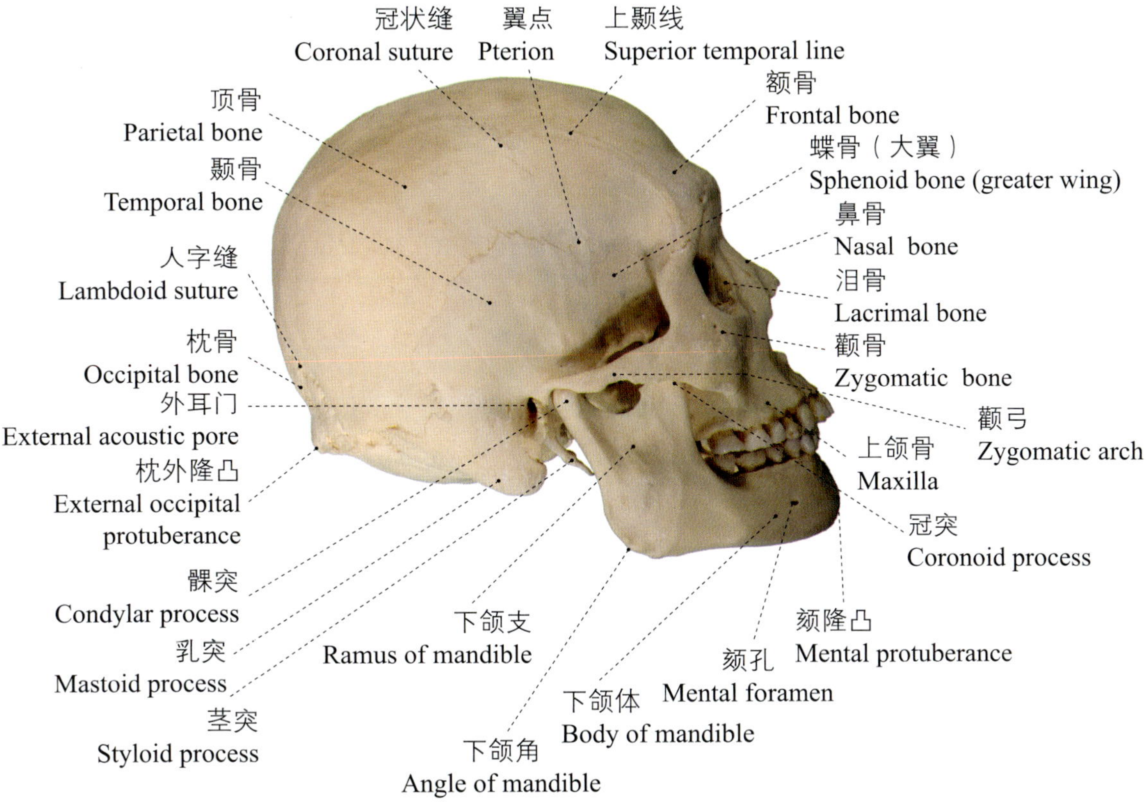

图 1–24　颅（外侧面观）

Skull. Lateral aspect

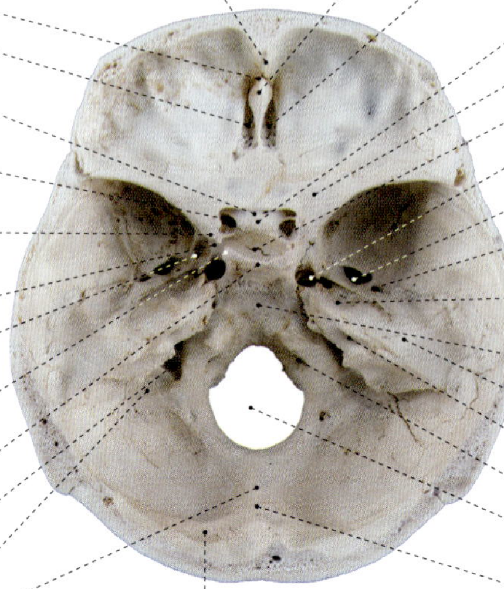

图 1–25　颅底内面

Internal surface of base of skull

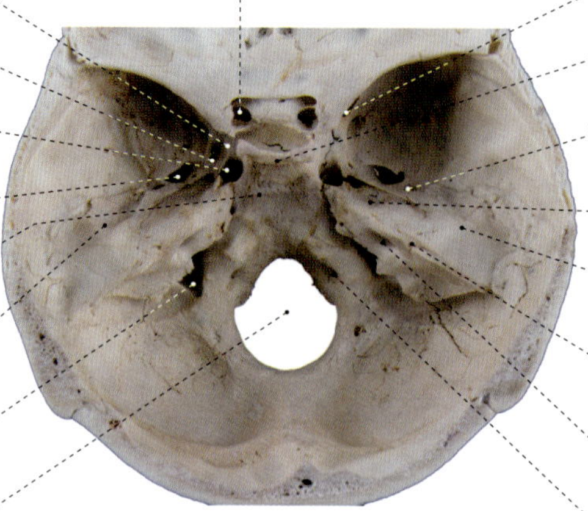

图 1–26　颅底内面（后上面观）

Internal surface of base of skull. Posterosuperior aspect

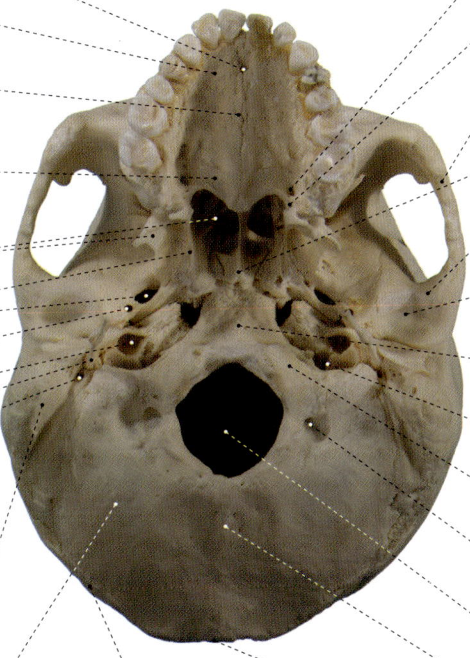

图 1–27　颅底外面

External surface of base of skull

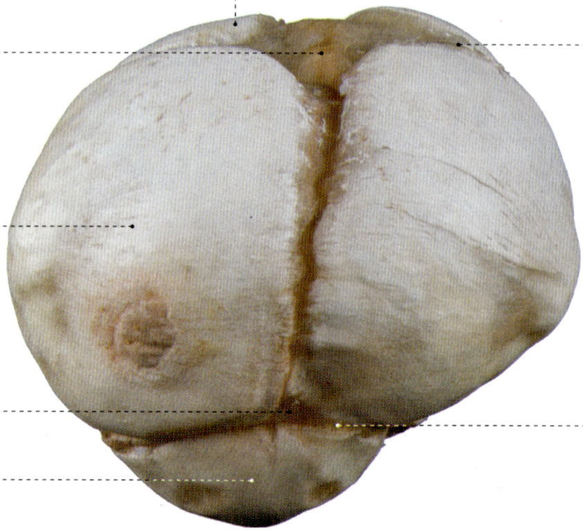

A. 上面观

Superior aspect

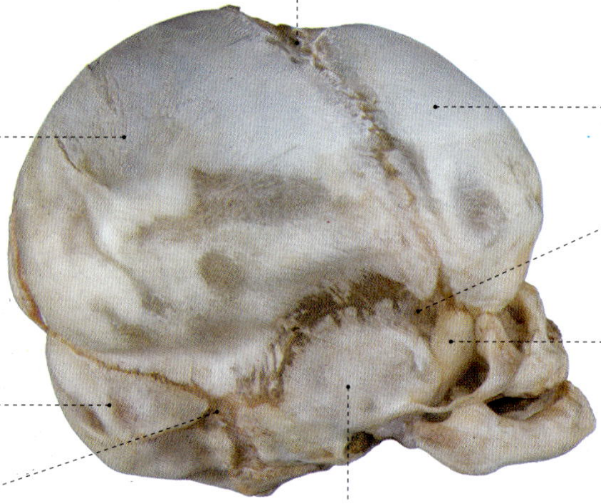

B. 外侧面观

Lateral aspect

图 1-28　新生儿颅

Skull of infant

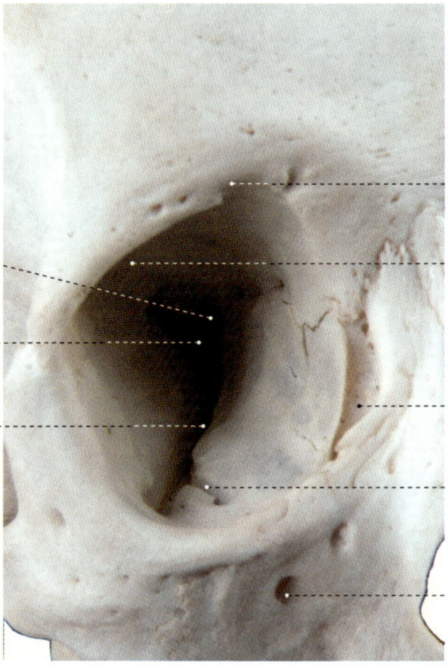

图 1–29　眶（前面观）
Orbit Anterior aspect

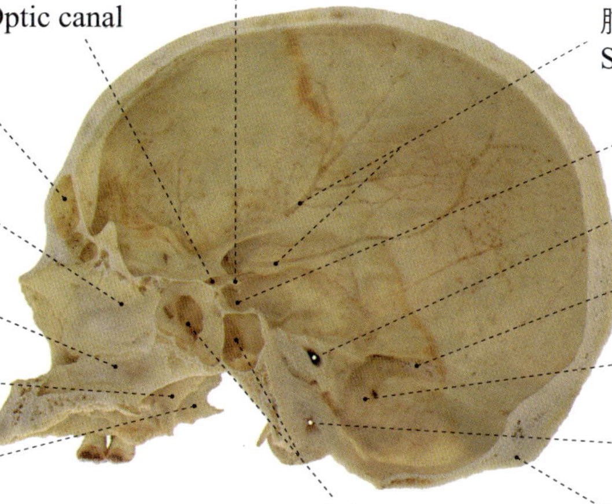

图 1–30　颅（矢状切面）
Skull. Sagittal section

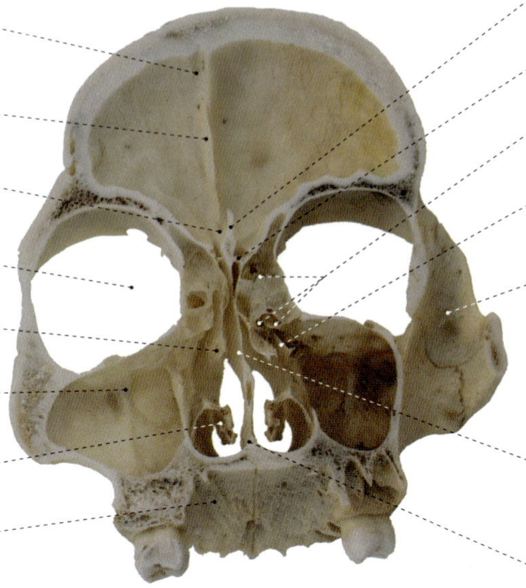

图 1–31　颅（冠状切面）（后面观）

Skull. Coronal section. Posterior aspect

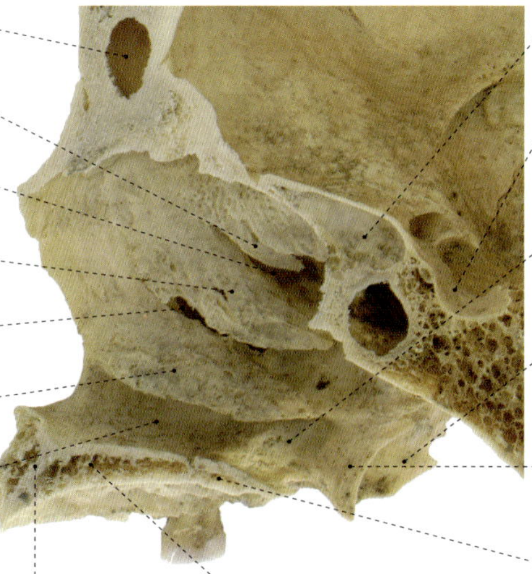

图 1–32　骨性鼻腔外侧壁 1

Lateral wall of the bony nasal cavity 1

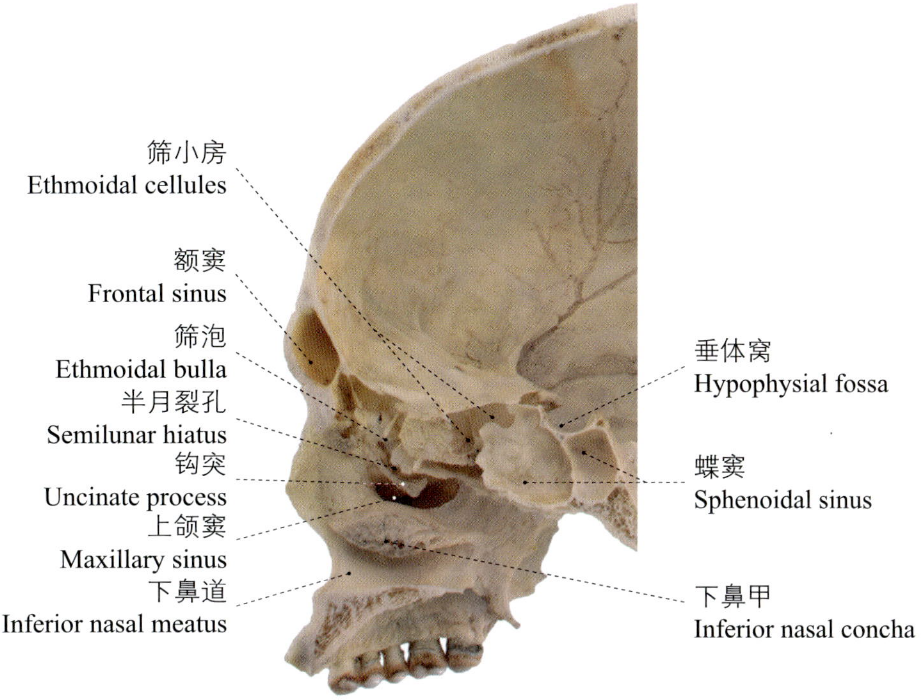

图 1–33　骨性鼻腔外侧壁 2

Lateral wall of the bony nasal cavity 2

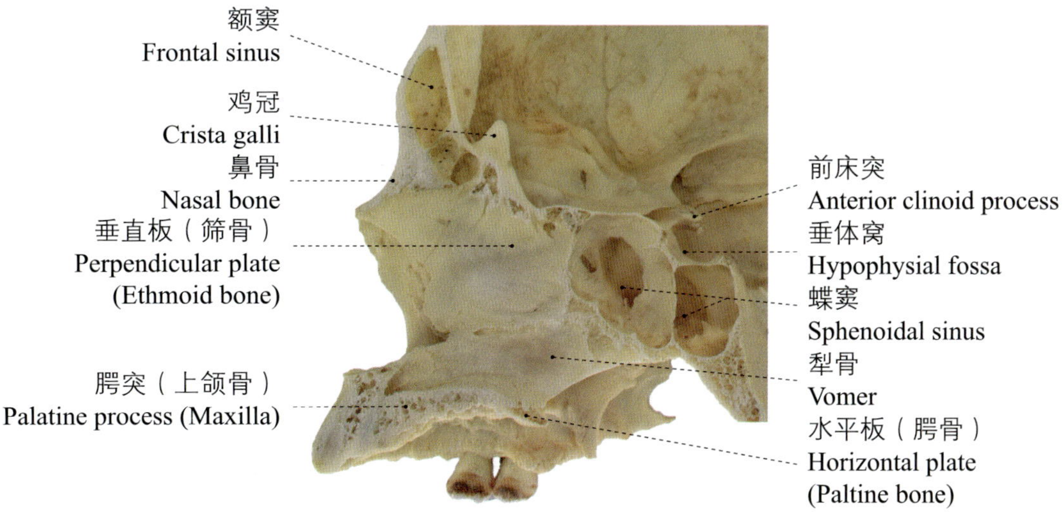

图 1–34　骨性鼻腔内侧壁

Medial wall of the bony nasal cavity

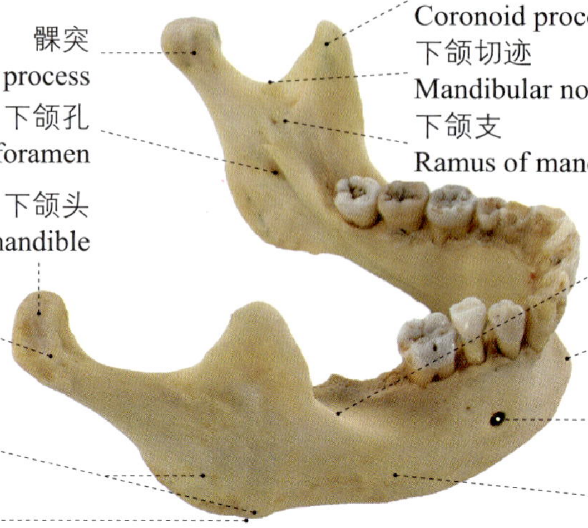

图 1–35　下颌骨（外侧面观）

Mandible. Lateral aspect

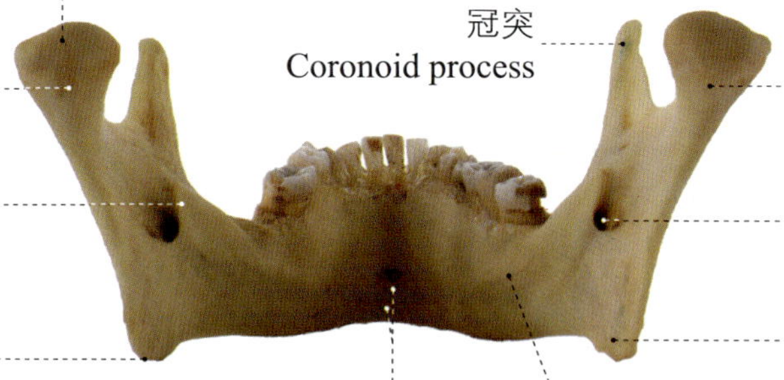

图 1–36　下颌骨（后面观）

Mandible. Posterior aspect

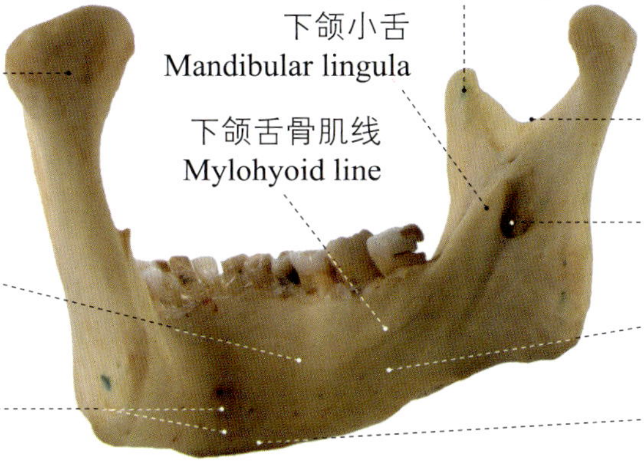

图 1–37　下颌骨（左后面观）

Mandible. Left posterior aspect

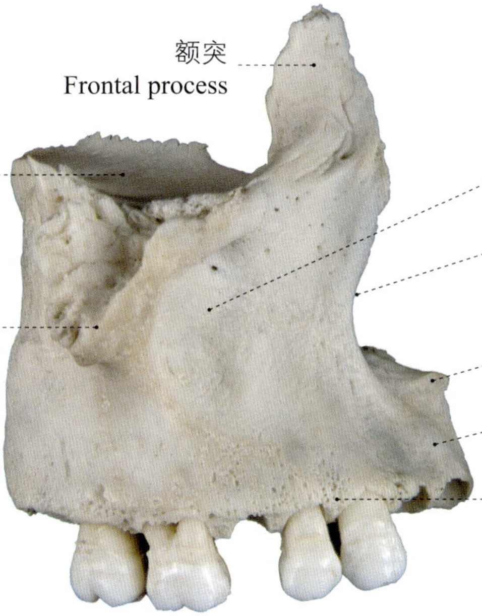

图 1–38　上颌骨（外侧面观）

Maxilla. Lateral aspect

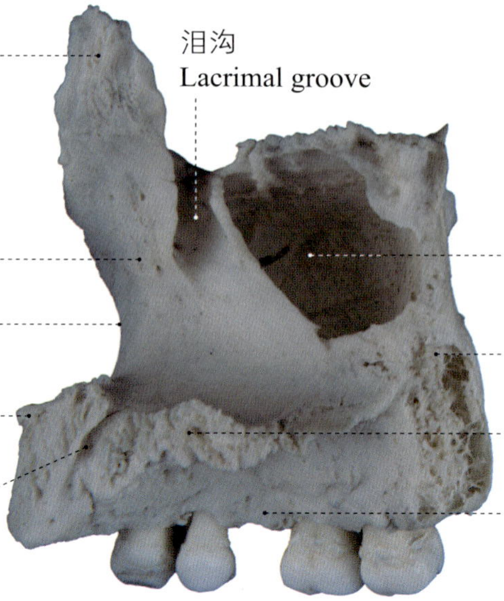

图 1-39　上颌骨（内侧面观）
Maxilla. Medial aspect

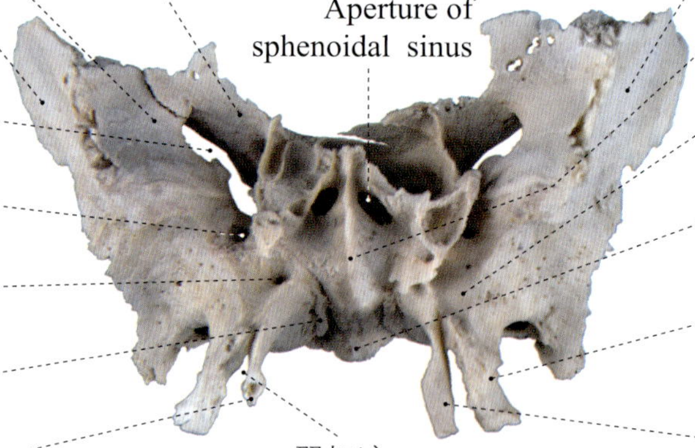

图 1-40　蝶骨（前面观）
Sphenoid bone. Anterior aspect

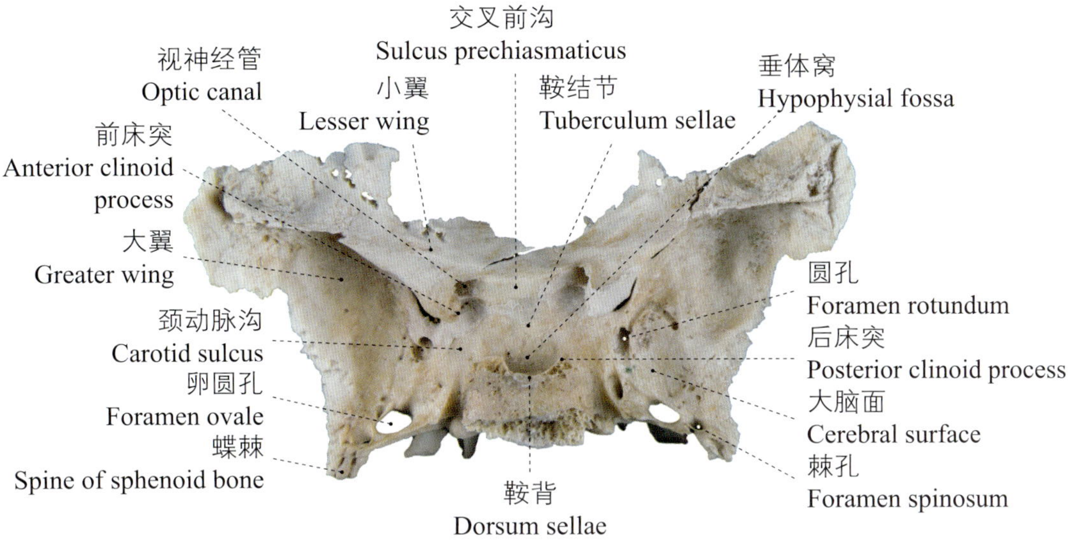

图 1–41　蝶骨（上面观）

Sphenoid bone. Superior aspect

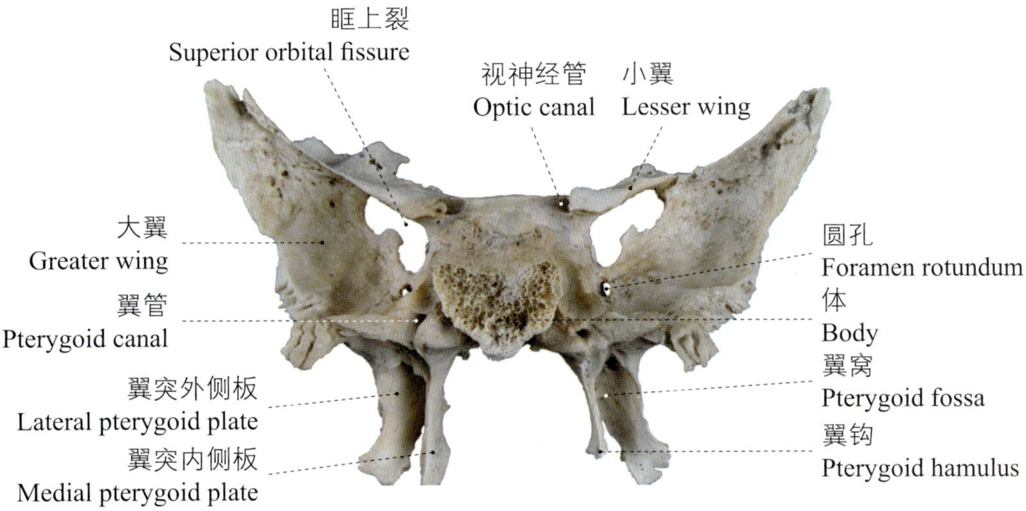

图 1–42　蝶骨（后面观）

Sphenoid bone. Posterior aspect

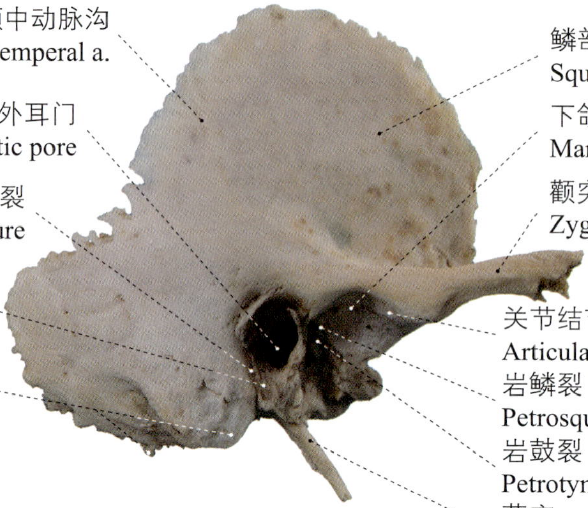

图 1–43　颞骨（外面观）

Temporal bone. External aspect

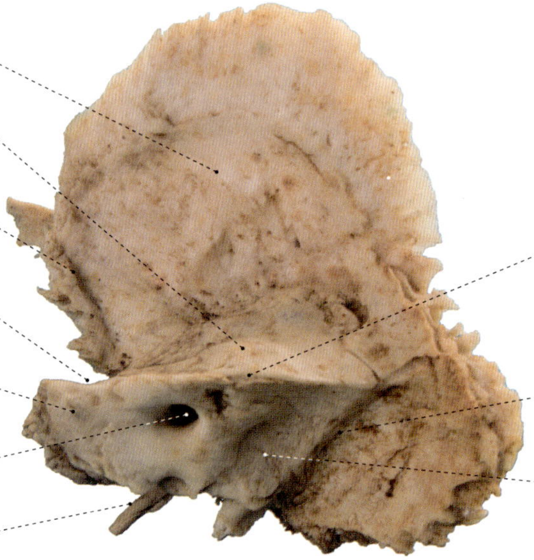

图 1–44　颞骨（内面观）

Temporal bone. Internal aspect

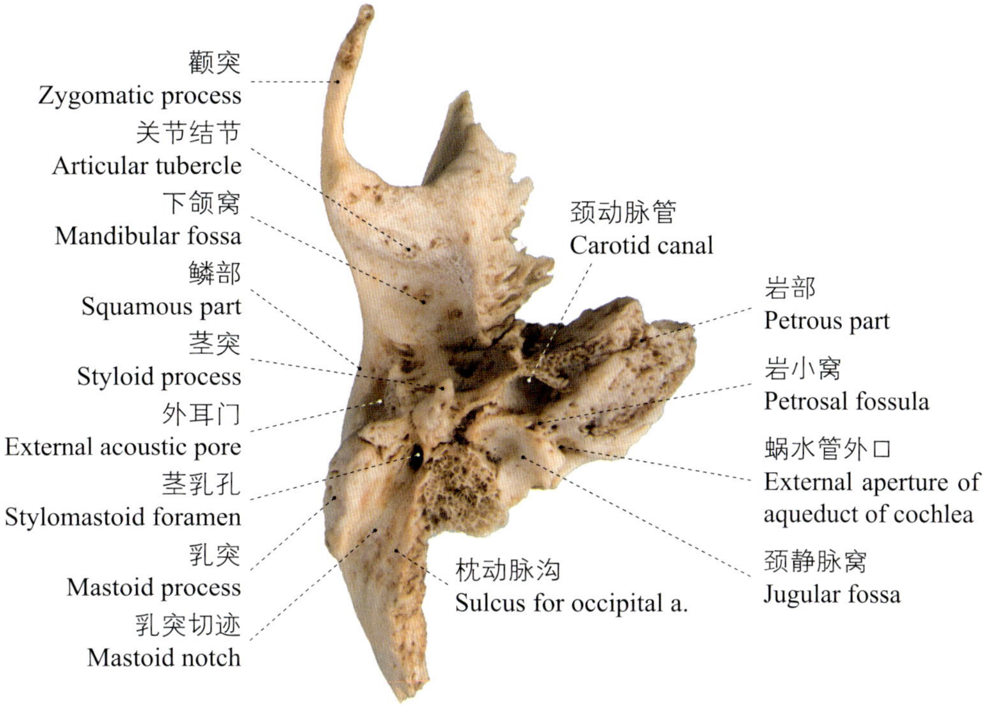

图 1-45 颞骨（下面观）
Temporal bone. Inferior aspect

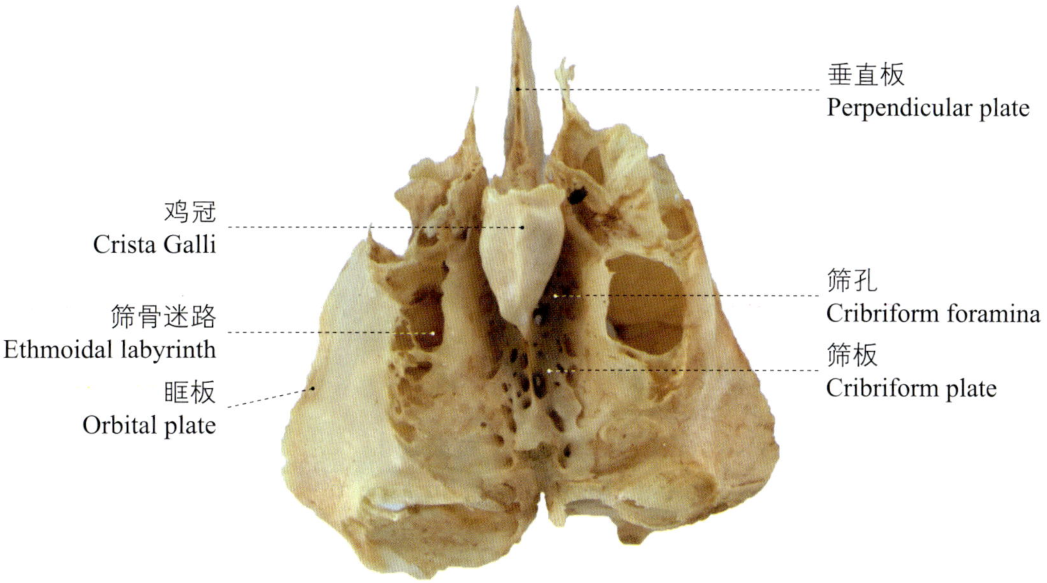

图 1-46 筛骨（上面观）
Ethmoid bone. Superior aspect

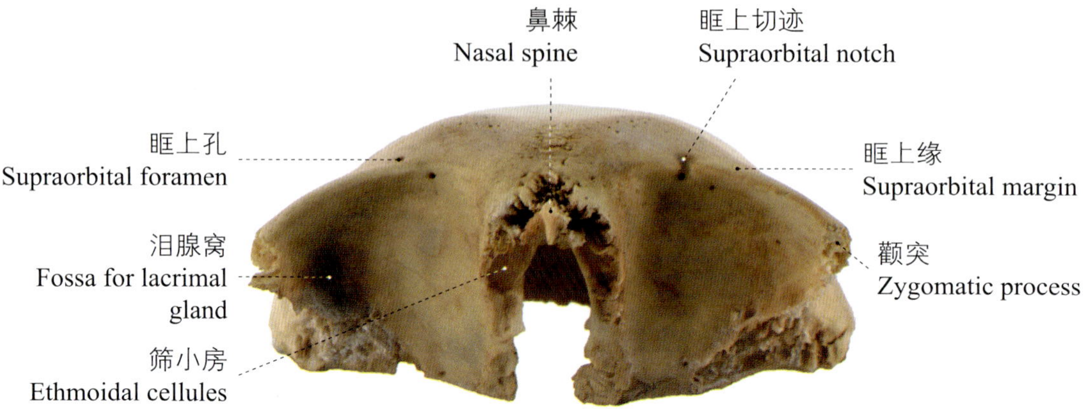

图 1–51　额骨（下面观）
Frontal bone. Inferior aspect

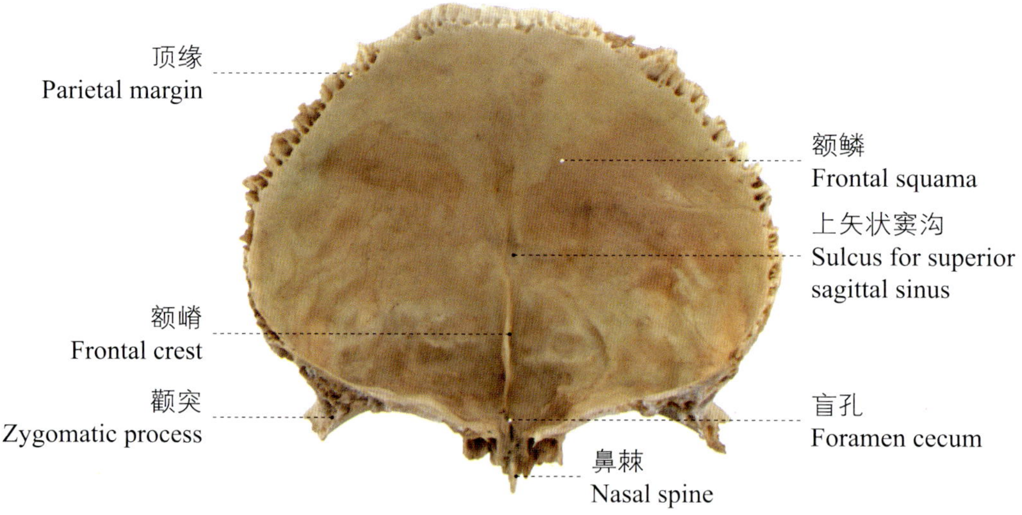

图 1–52　额骨（内面观）
Frontal bone. Internal aspect

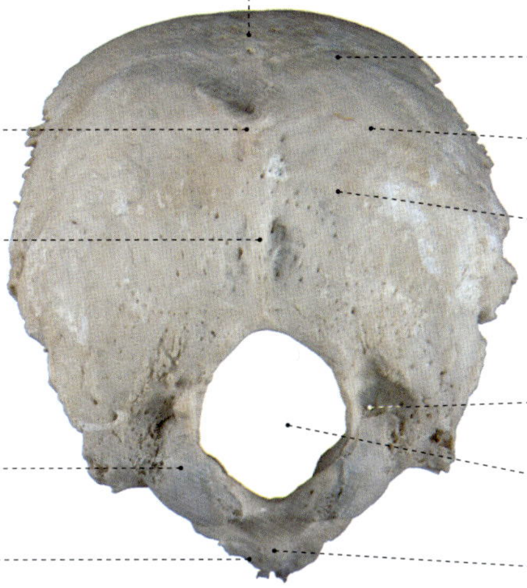

图 1–53　枕骨（外面观）

Occipital bone. External aspect

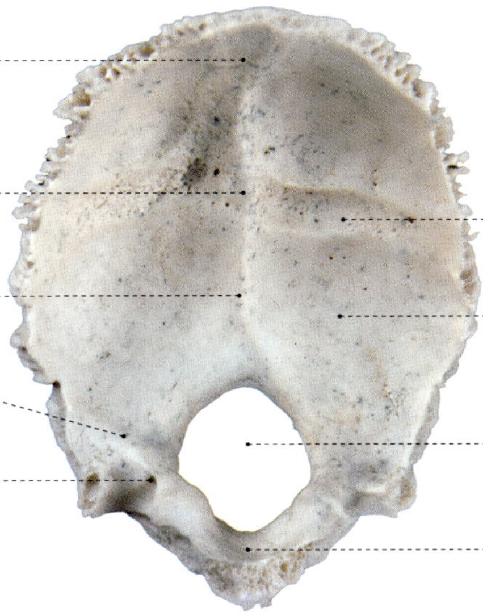

图 1–54　枕骨（内面观）

Occipital bone. Internal aspect

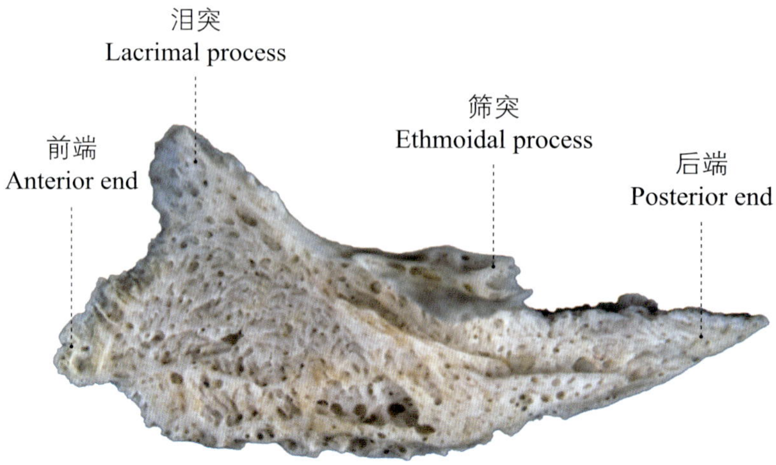

图 1–55　下鼻甲（内侧面观）
Inferior nasal concha. Medial aspect

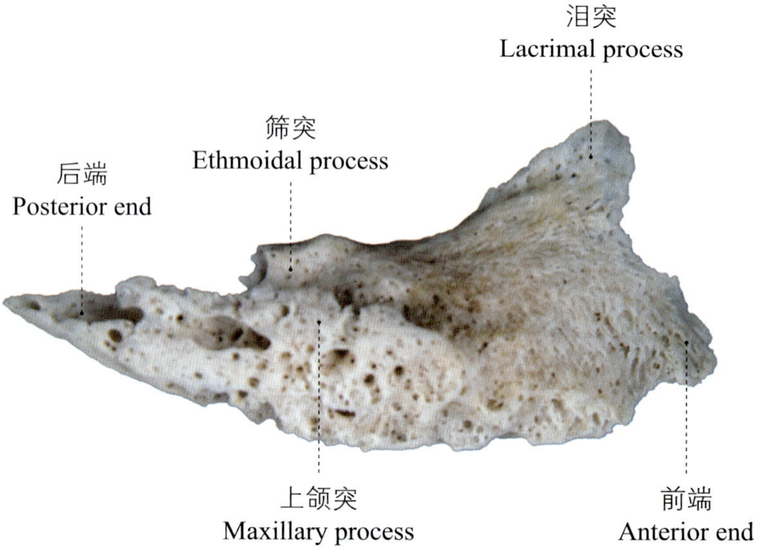

图 1–56　下鼻甲（外侧面观）
Inferior nasal concha.Lateral aspect

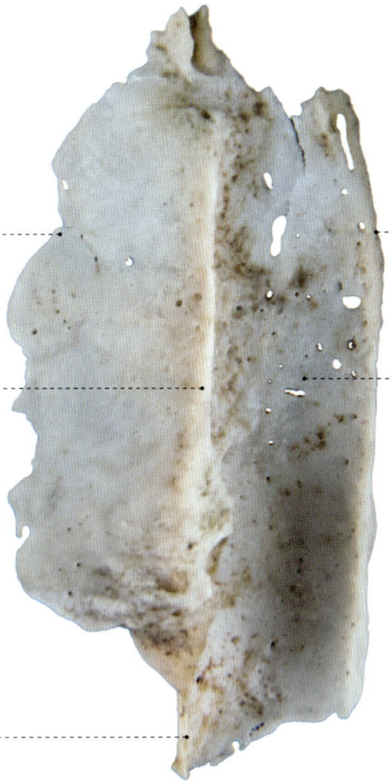

图 1–57 泪骨（外侧面观）
Lacrimal bone. Lateral aspect

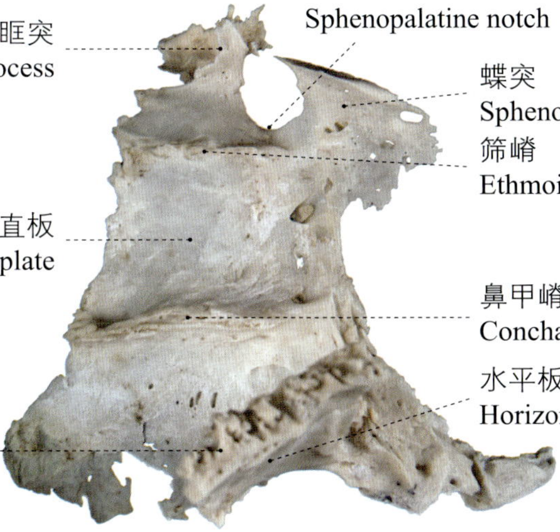

图 1–58 腭骨（内侧面观）
Palatine bone. Medial aspect

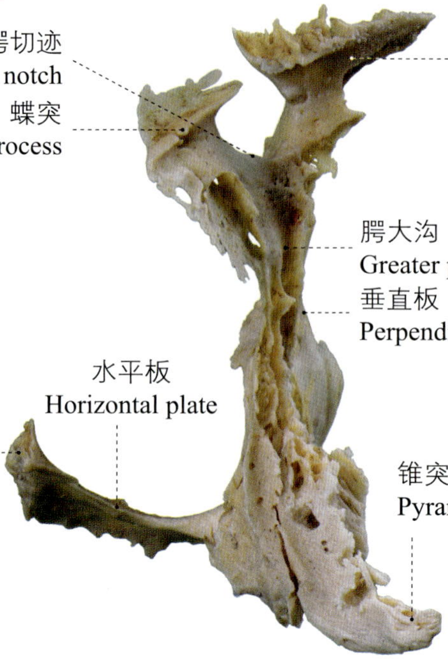

图 1–59　腭骨（后面观）

Palatine bone. Posterior aspect

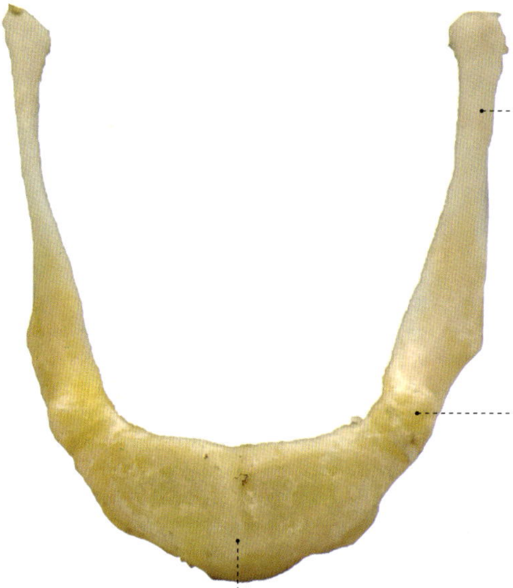

图 1–60　舌骨（上面观）

Hyoid bone. Superior aspect

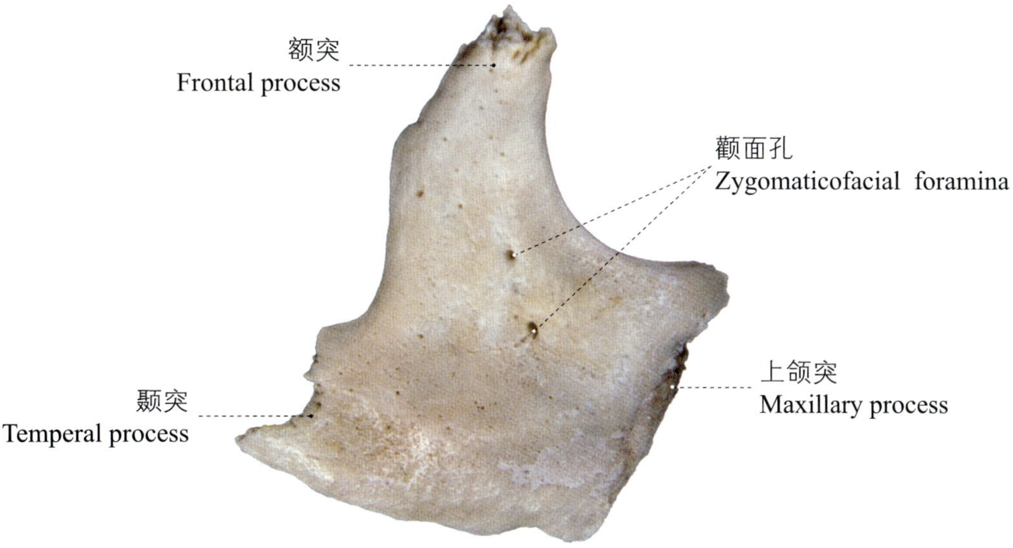

图 1–61　颧骨（外侧面观）
Zygomatic bone. Lateral aspect

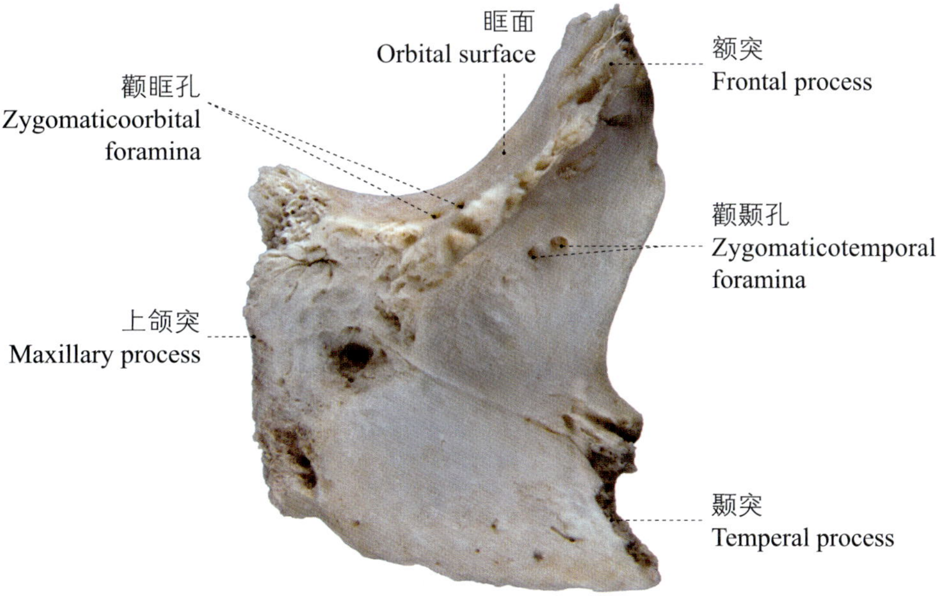

图 1–62　颧骨（内侧面观）
Zygomatic bone. Medial aspect

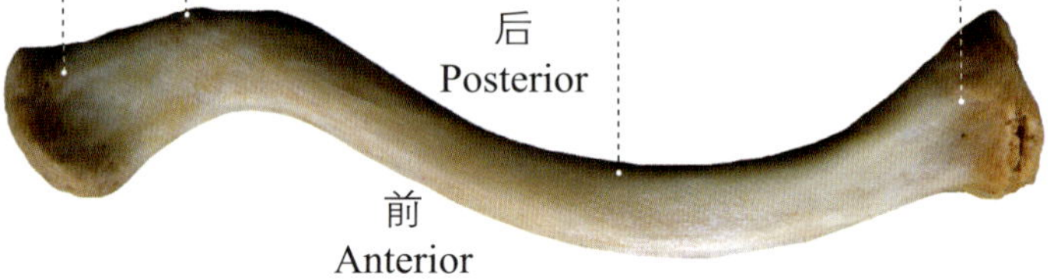

图 1–63 锁骨（上面观）
Clavicle. Superior aspect

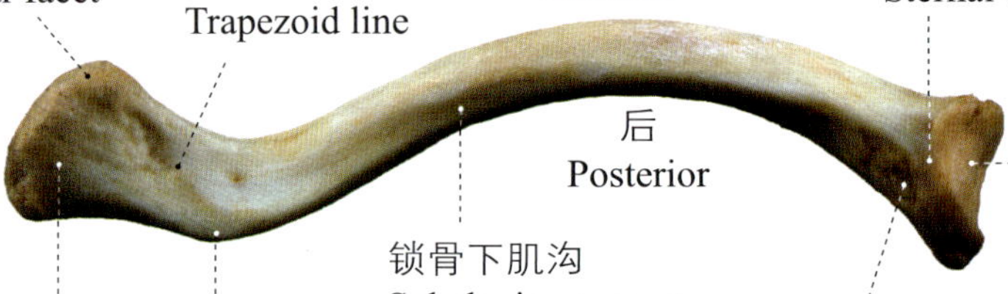

图 1–64 锁骨（下面观）
Clavicle. Inferior aspect

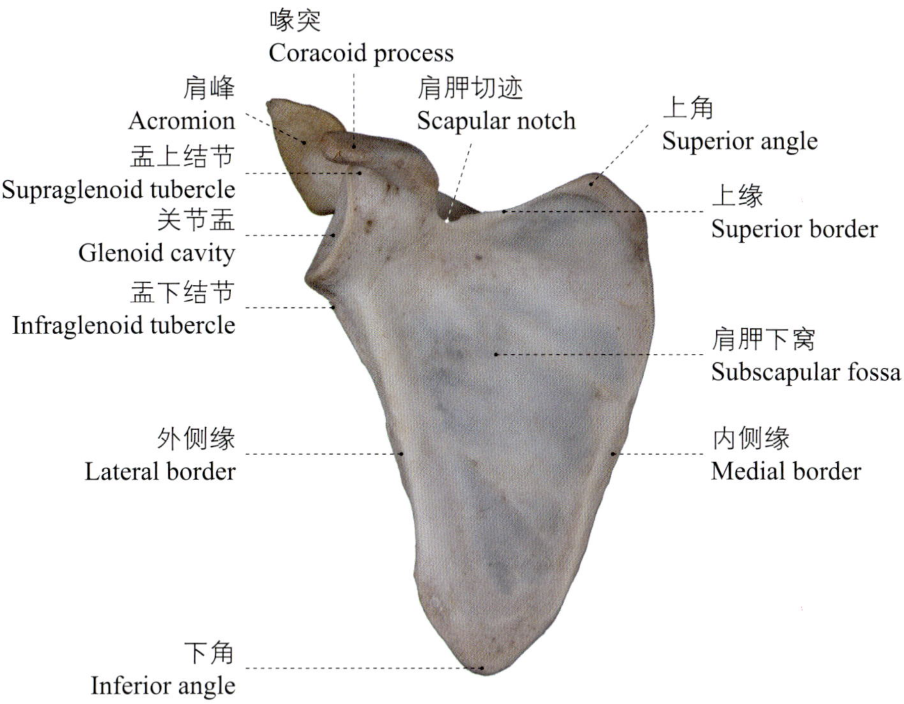

图 1–65 肩胛骨（前面观）
Scapula. Anterior aspect

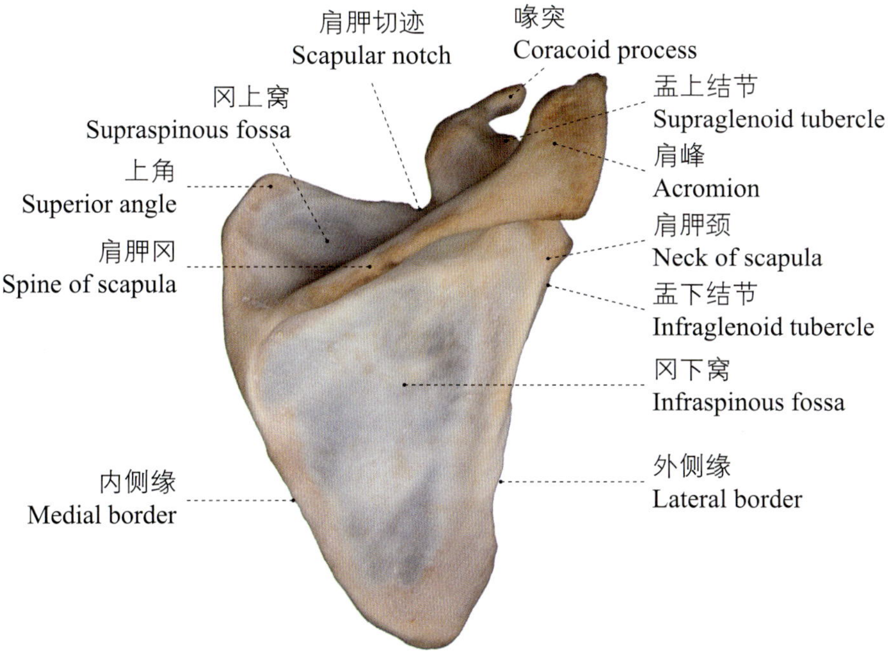

图 1–66 肩胛骨（后面观）
Scapula. Posterior aspect

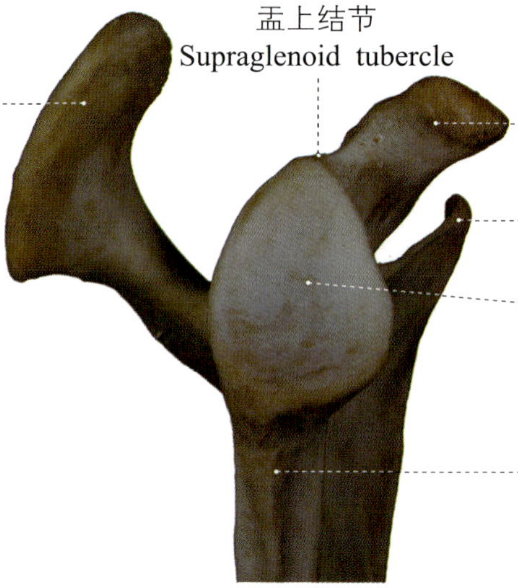

图 1–67　肩胛骨（外侧面观）
Scapula. Lateral aspect

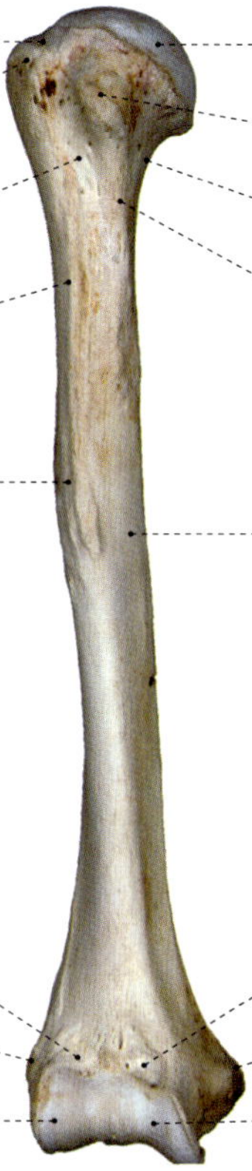

图 1–68　肱骨（前面观）
Humerus. Anterior aspect

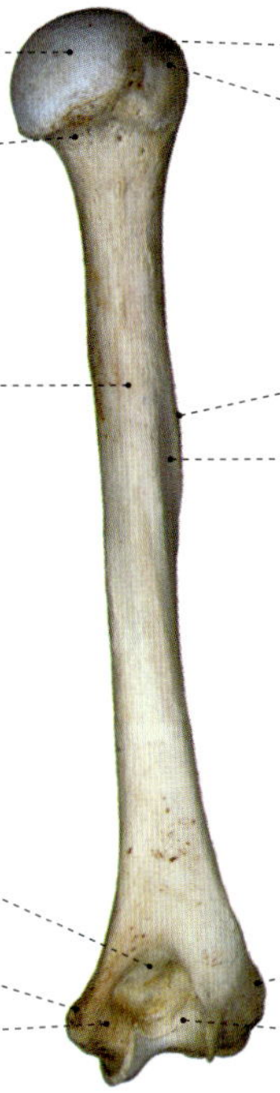

图 1–69　肱骨（后面观）

Humerus. Posterior aspect

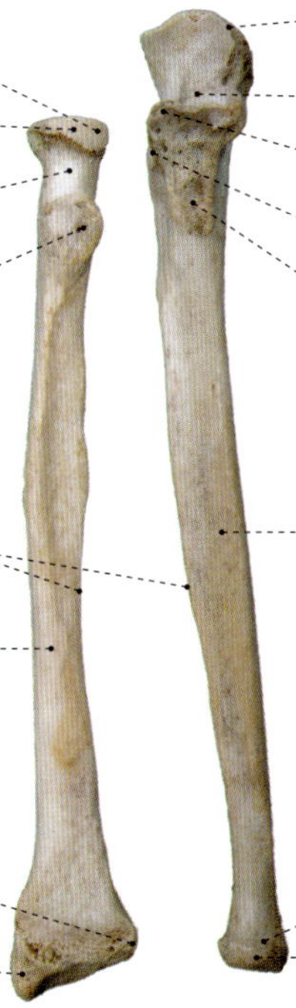

图 1–70　桡骨和尺骨（前面观）

Radius and ulna. Anterior aspect

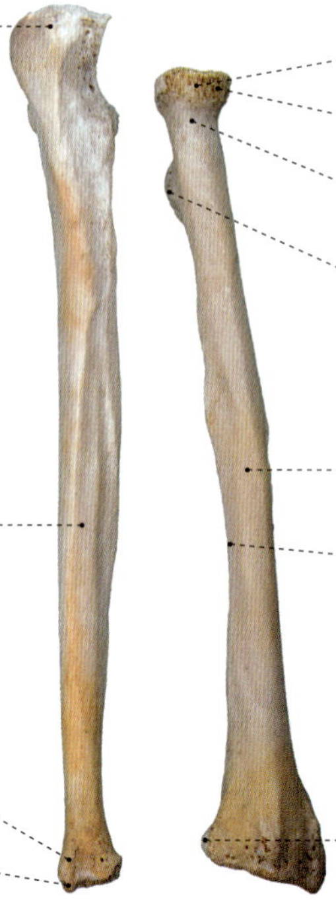

图 1–71　桡骨和尺骨（后面观）

Radius and ulna.Posterior aspect

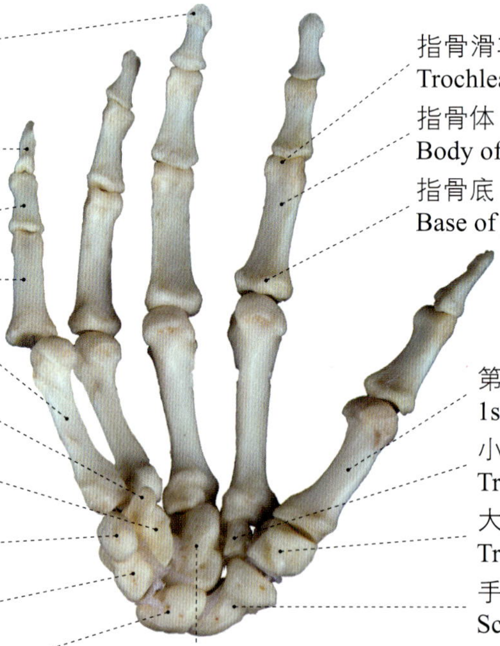

图 1–72　手骨（前面观）

Bones of the hand. Anterior aspect

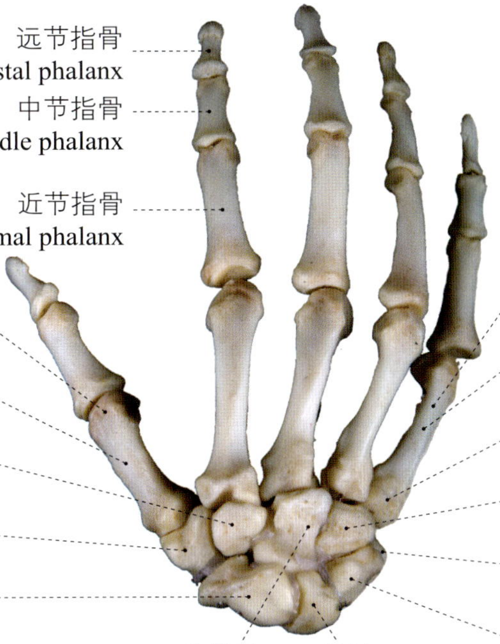

图 1–73 手骨（后面观）

Bones of the hand. Posterior aspect

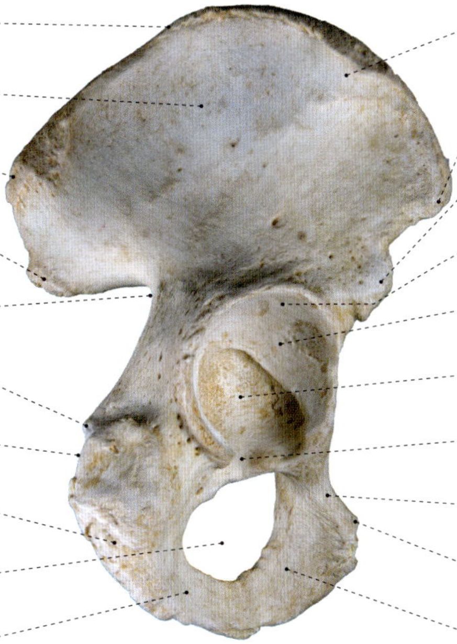

图 1–74 髋骨（外面观）

Hip bone. External aspect

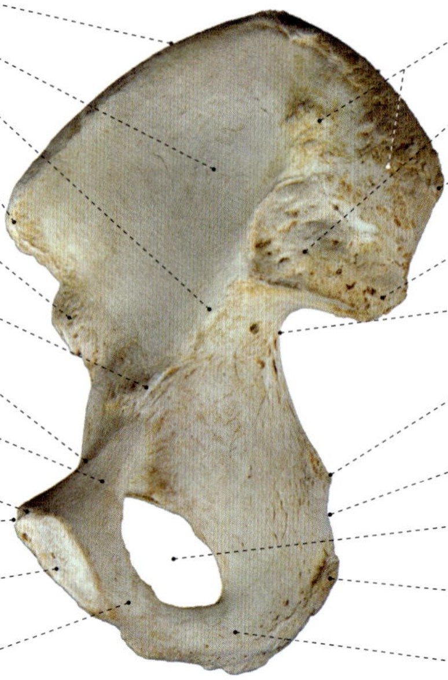

图 1–75 髋骨（内面观）
Hip bone. Internal aspect

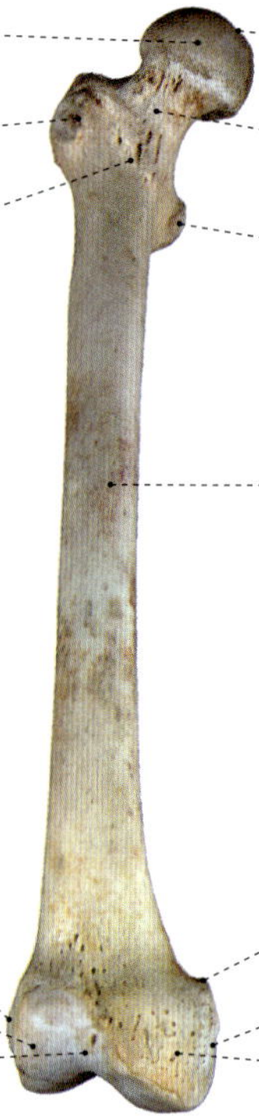

图 1–76 股骨（前面观）
Femur. Anterior aspect

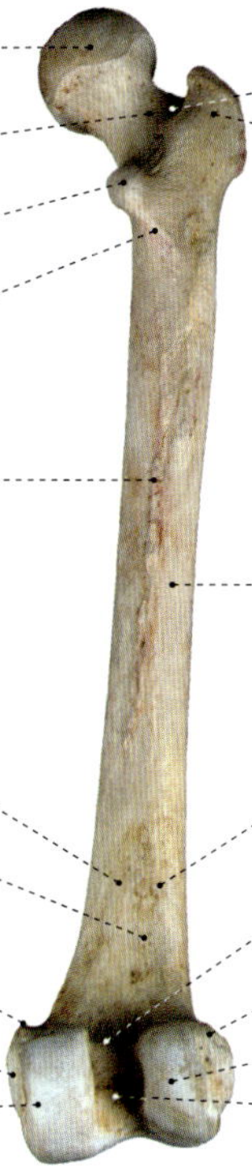

图 1–77　股骨（后面观）

Femur. Posterior aspect

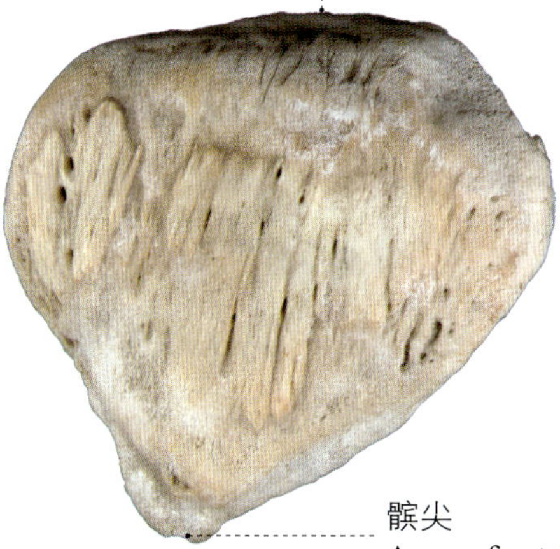

图 1–78　髌骨（前面观）

Patella. Anterior aspect

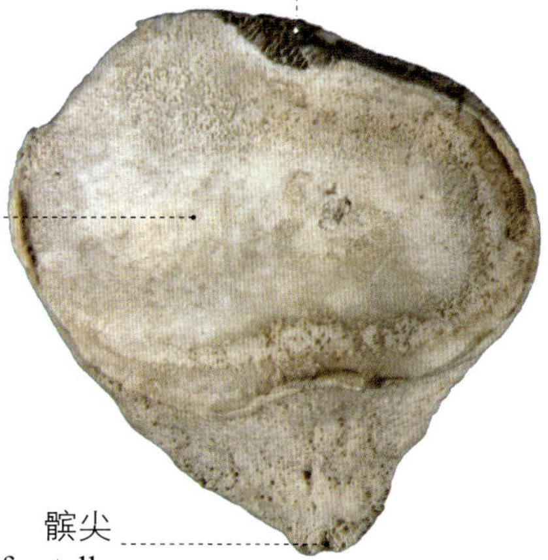

图 1–79　髌骨（后面观）

Patella. Posterior aspect

第二节　骨连接

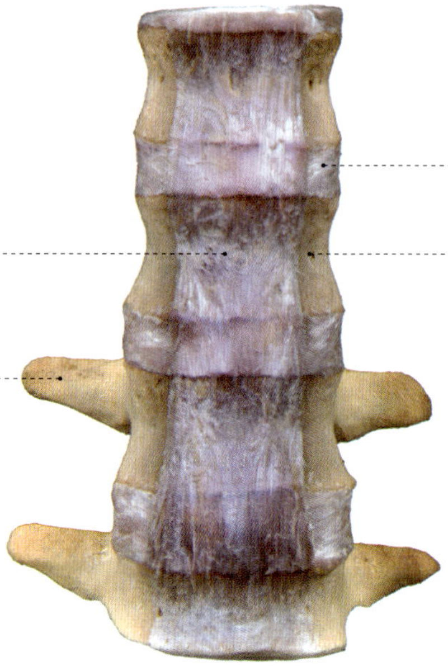

图 1-84　椎骨间的连结（前面观）
Intervertebral joints. Anterior aspect

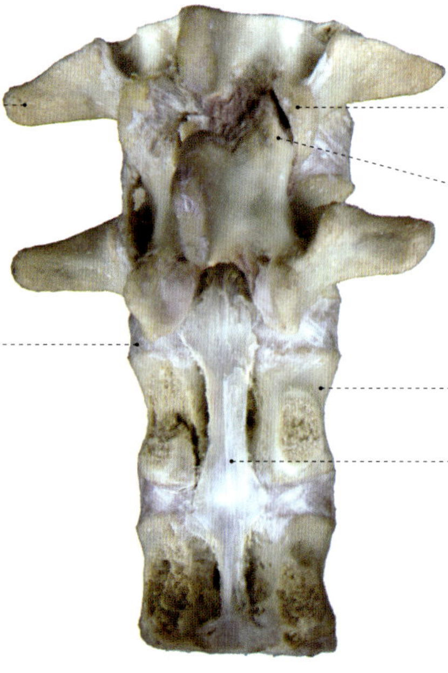

图 1-85　椎骨间的连结（后面观）
Intervertebral joints. Posterior aspect

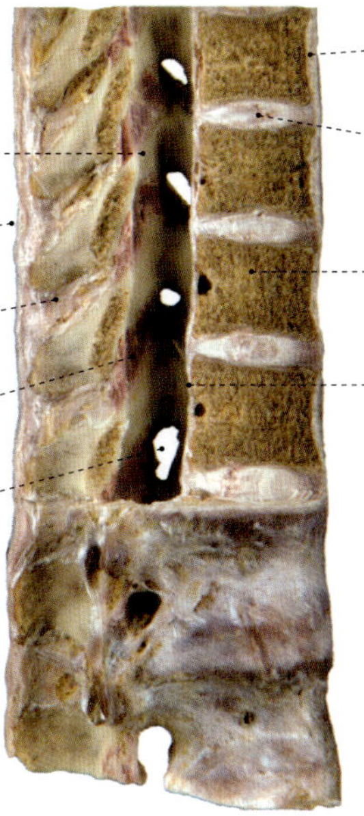

图 1–86　椎骨间的连结（正中矢状切面）
Intervertebral joints. Median sagittal section

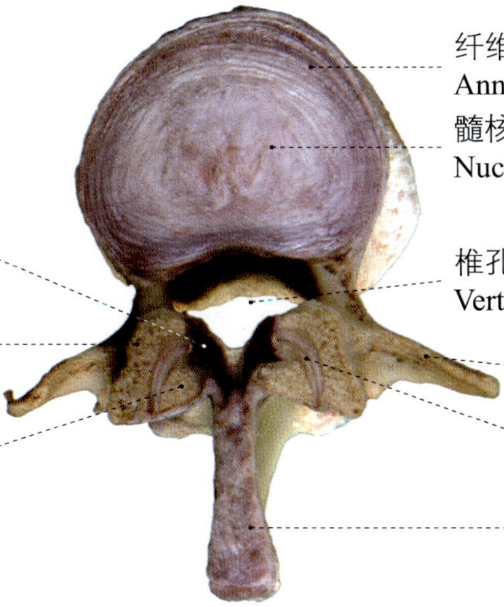

图 1–87　椎间盘（下面观）
Intervertebral disc. Inferior aspect

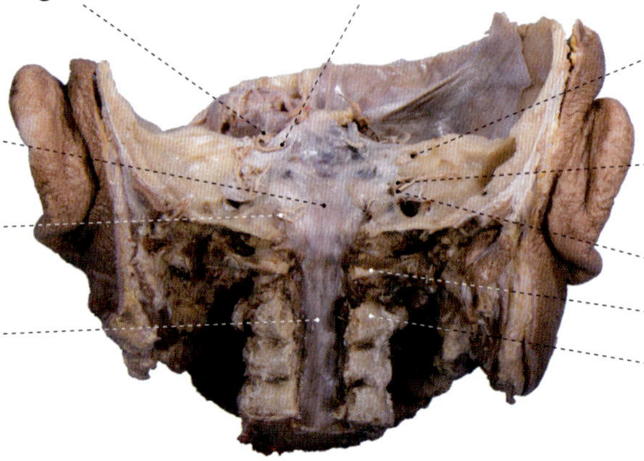

图 1-88　寰枕和寰枢关节（后面观）（1）

Atlantooccipital and atlantoaxial joint. Posterior aspect (1)

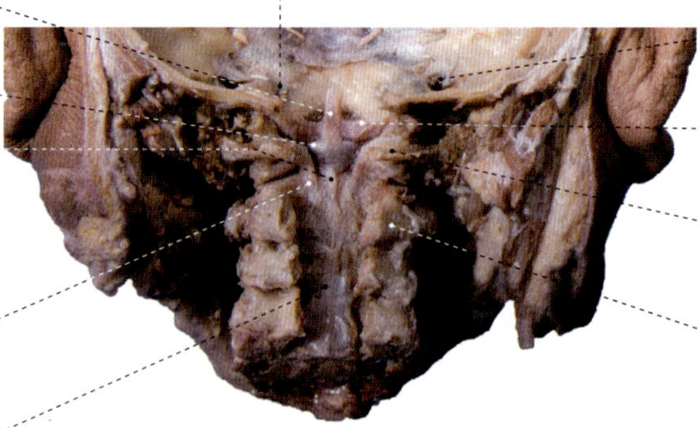

图 1-89　寰枕和寰枢关节（后面观）（2）

Atlantooccipital and atlantoaxial joint. Posterior aspect (2)

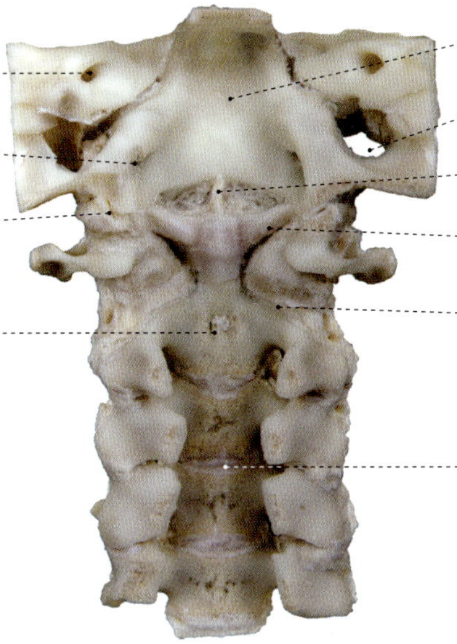

图 1–90　寰枕和寰枢关节（后面观）（3）
Atlantooccipital and atlantoaxial joint. Posterior aspect (3)

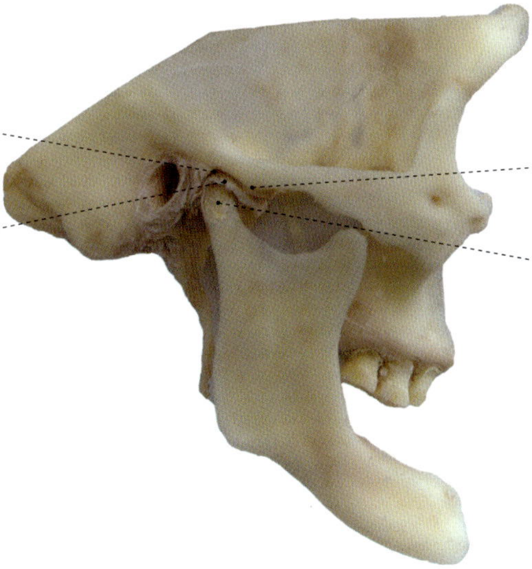

图 1–91　颞下颌关节（外侧面观）
Temporomandibular joint. Lateral aspect

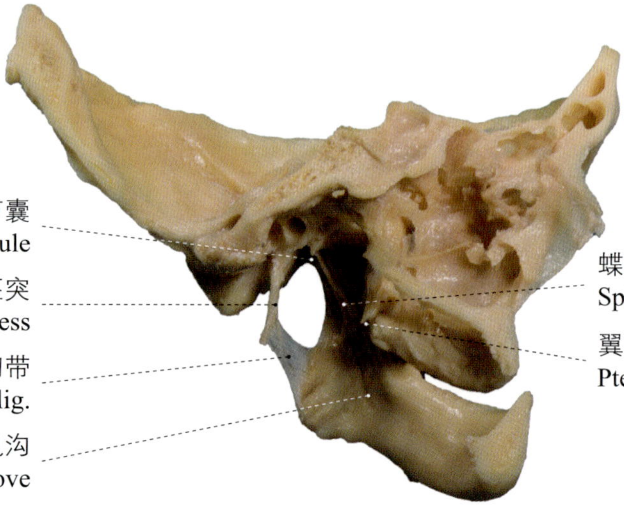

图 1–92　颞下颌关节（内侧面观）

Temporomandibular joint. Medial aspect

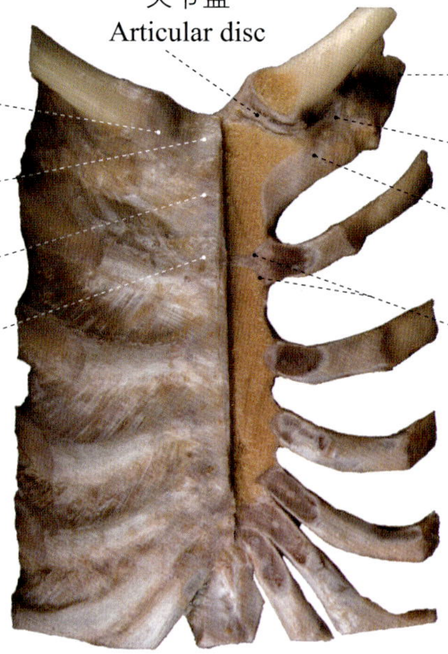

图 1–93　胸锁关节和胸肋关节（前面观）

Sternoclavicular and sternocostal joints . Anterior aspect

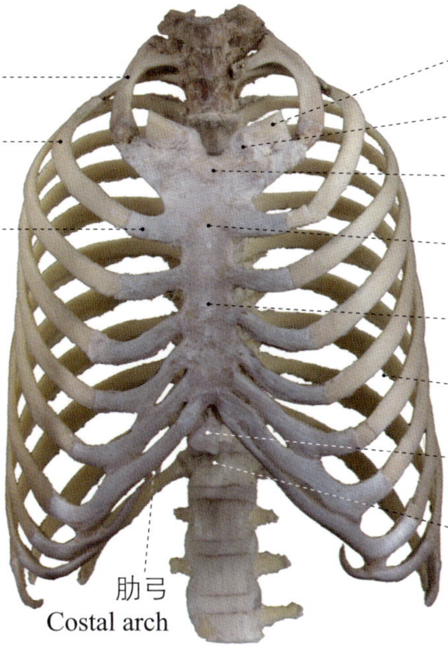

图 1–94　胸廓（前面观）

Thorax. Anterior aspect

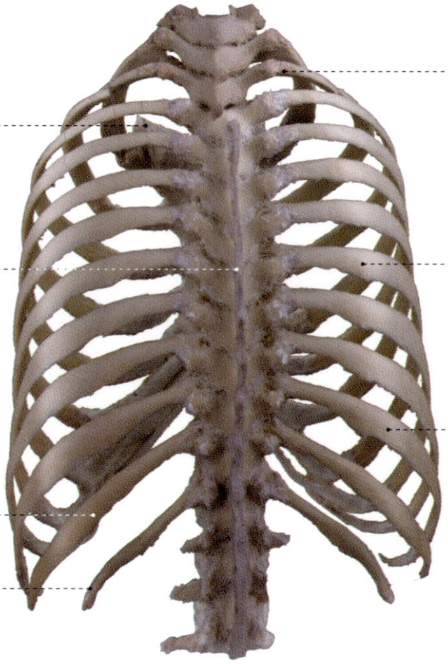

图 1–95　胸廓（后面观）

Thorax. Posterior aspect

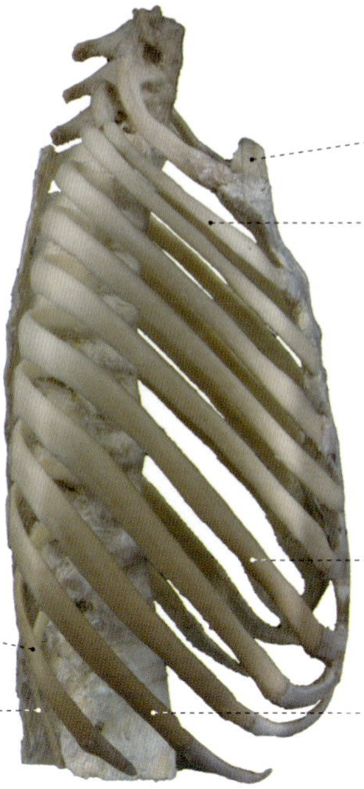

图 1–96　胸廓（外侧面观）
Thorax. Lateral aspect

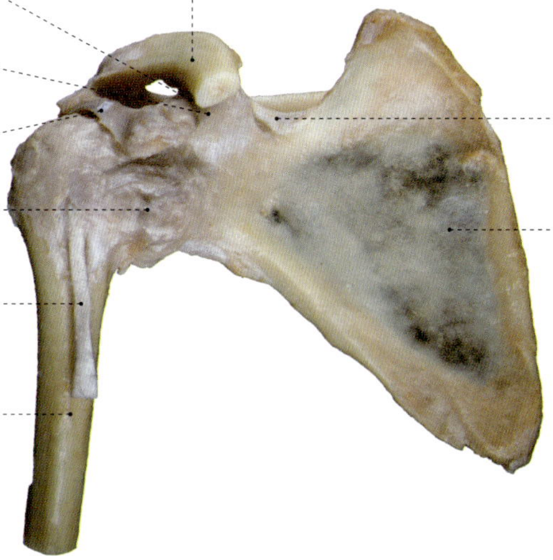

图 1–97　肩关节（前面观）
Shoulder joint. Anterior aspect

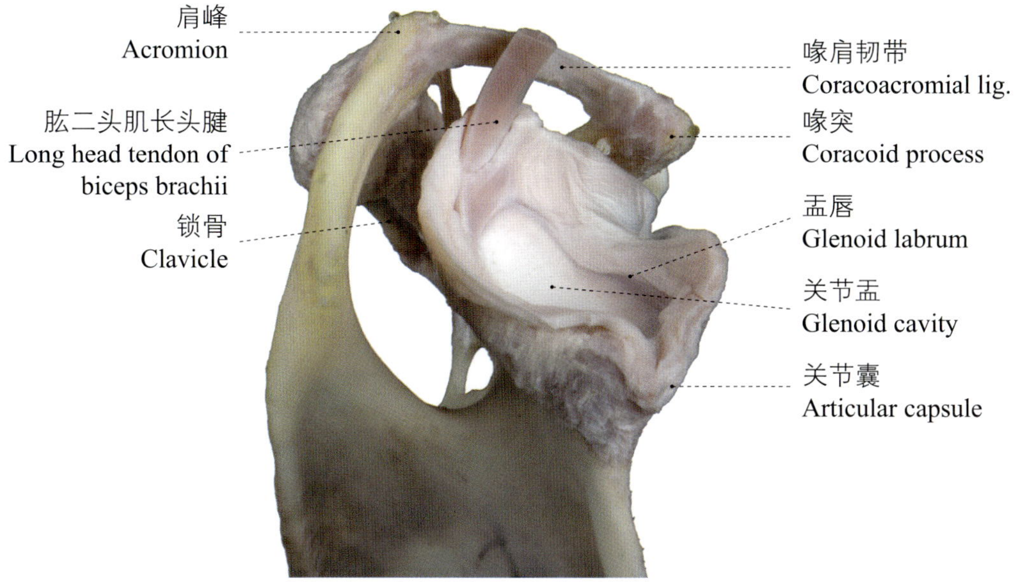

图 1–98 肩关节（内面观）
Shoulder joint. Internal aspect

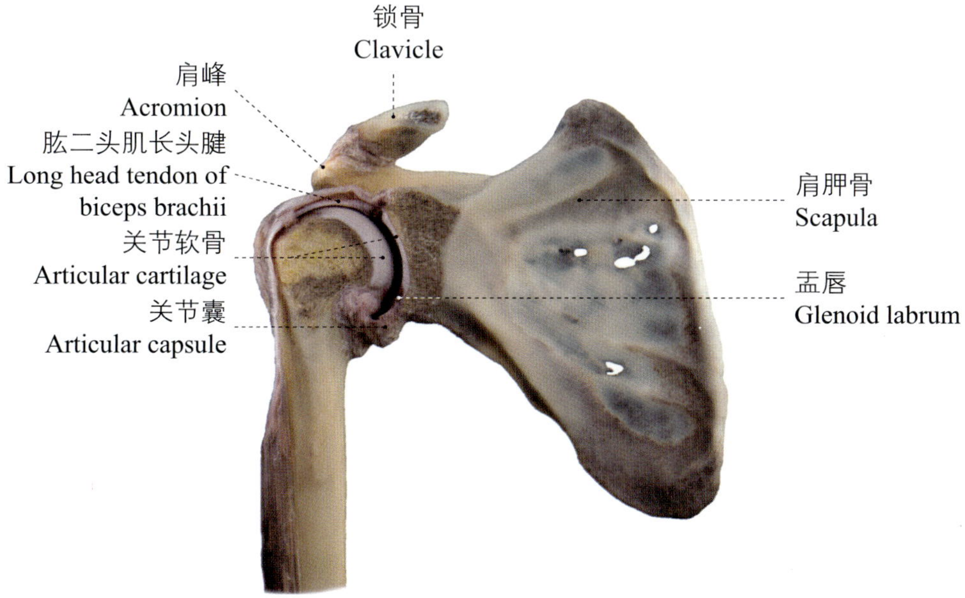

图 1–99 肩关节（冠状切面）
Shoulder joint. Coronal section

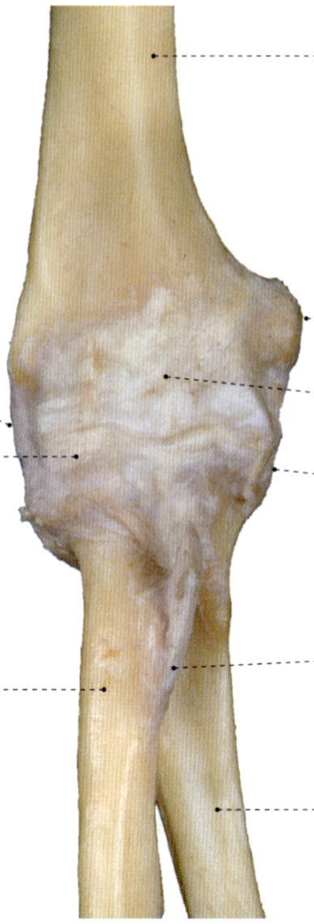

图 1–100　肘关节（前面观）

Elbow joint. Anterior aspect

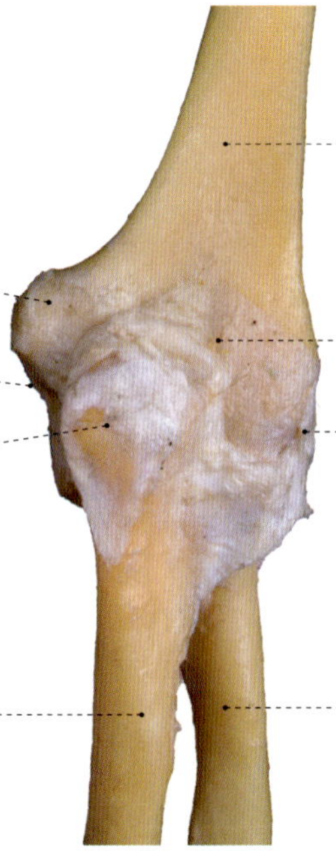

图 1–101　肘关节（后面观）

Elbow joint. Posterior aspect

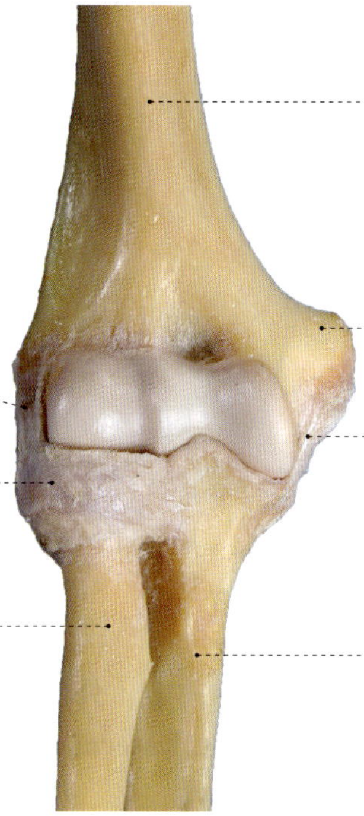

图 1–102　肘关节（前面观，打开关节囊）
Elbow joint. Anterior aspect, opened articular capsule

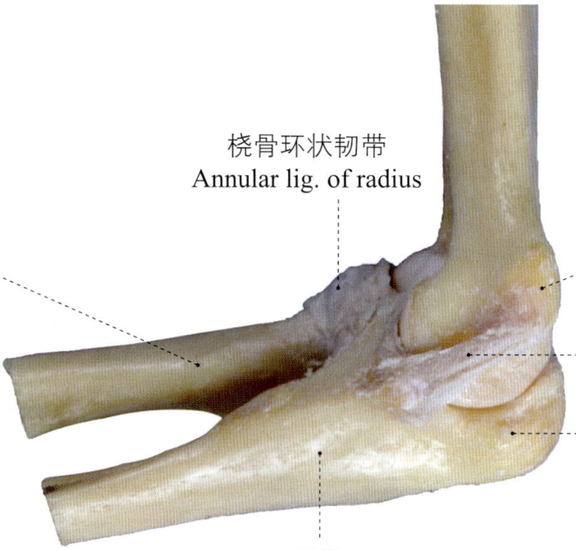

图 1–103　肘关节（内侧面观）
Elbow joint. Medial aspect

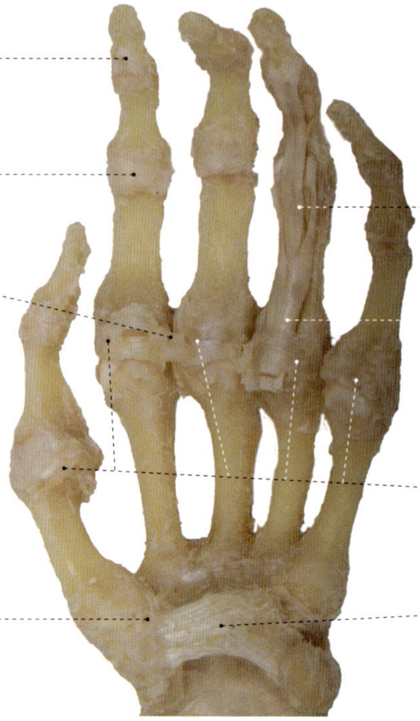

图 1–108　手关节（前面观）

Joints of hand. Anterior aspect

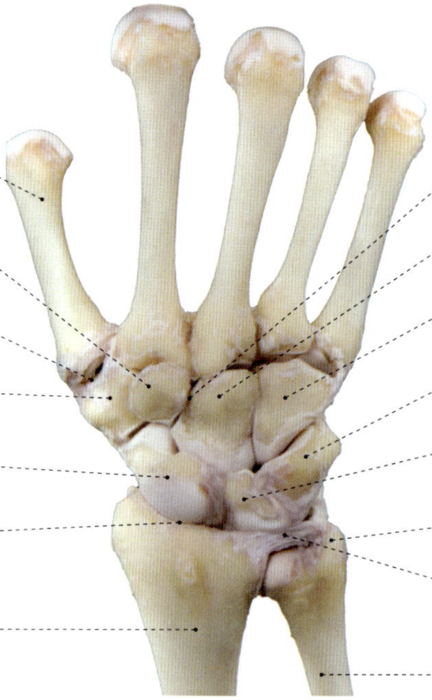

图 1–109　手关节（后面观）

Joints of hand. Posterior aspect

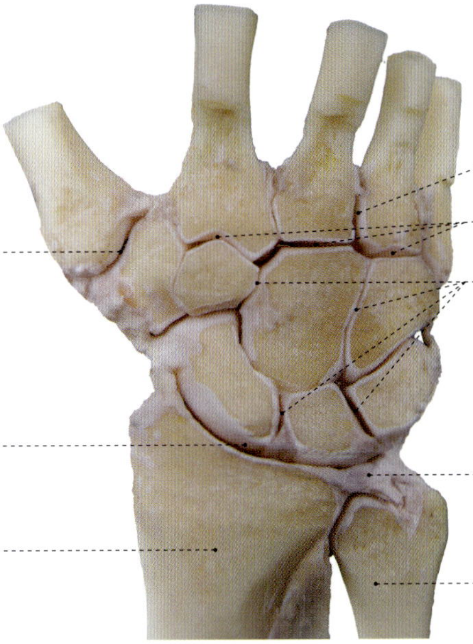

图 1–110　手关节的冠状切面（后面观）

Coronal section of Joints of hand. Posterior aspect

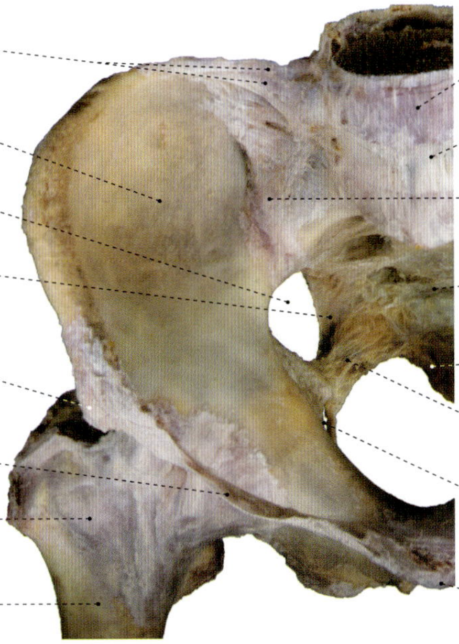

图 1–111　骨盆的连结（前面观）

Articulations of pelvis. Anterior aspect

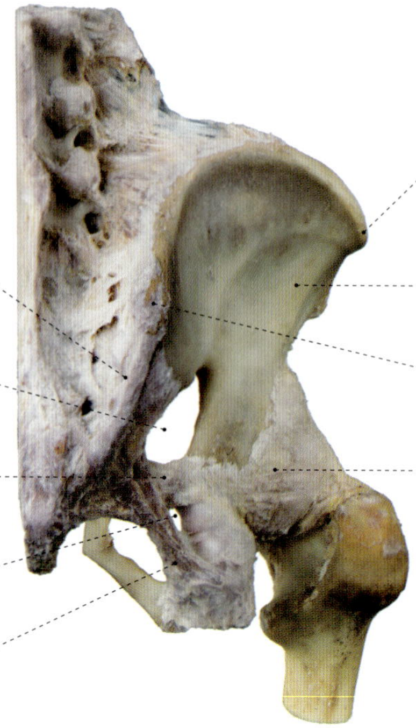

图 1–112　骨盆的连结（后面观）
Articulations of pelvis. Posterior aspect

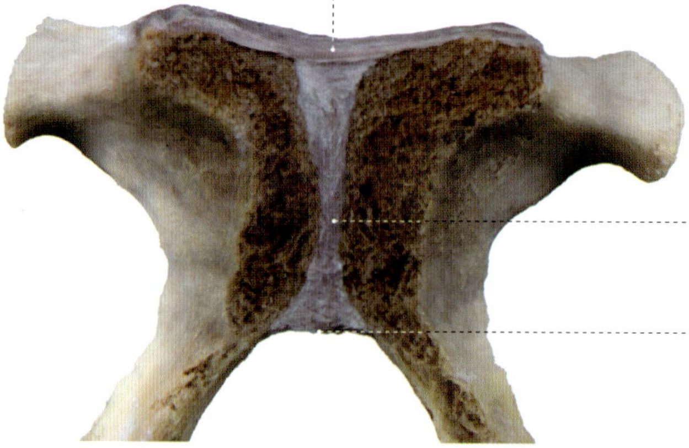

图 1–113　耻骨联合（冠状切面）
Pubic symphysis. Coronal aspect

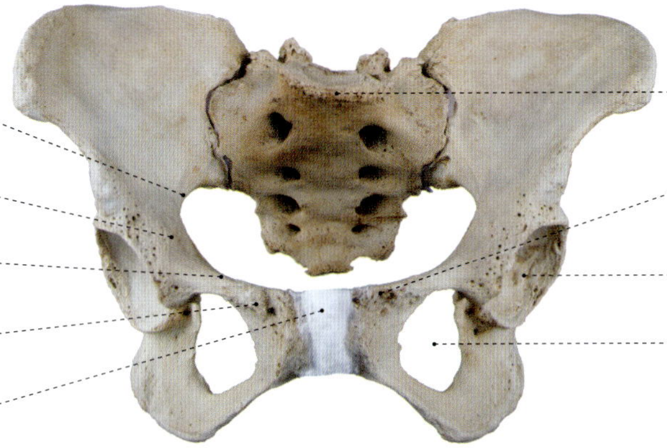

图 1-114　骨盆（女性）
Female pelvis

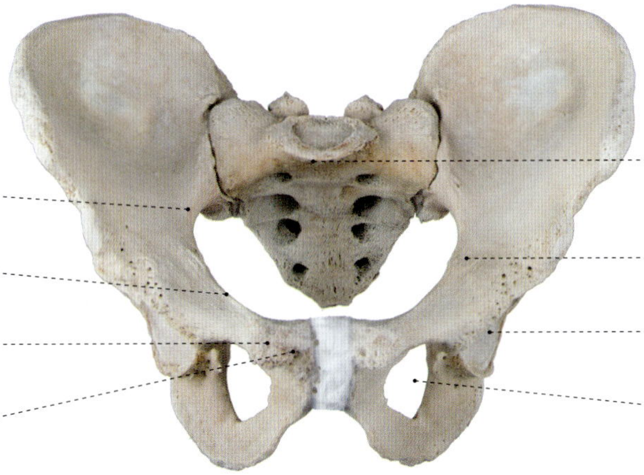

图 1-115　骨盆（男性）
Male pelvis

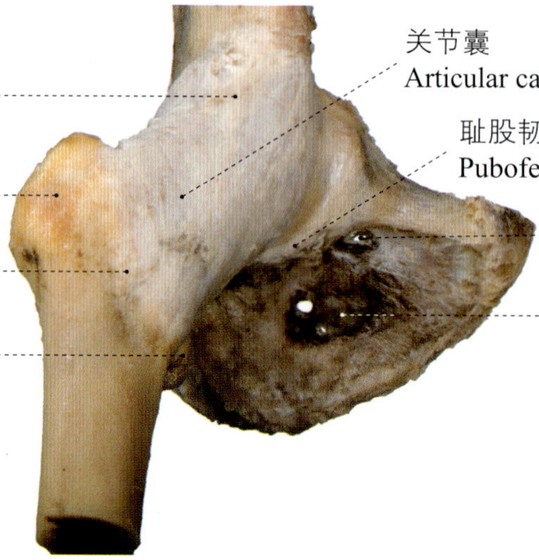

图 1–116　髋关节（前面观）
Hip joint. Anterior aspect

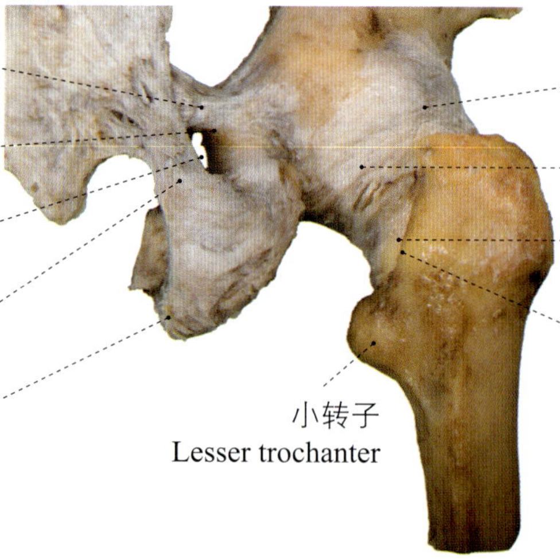

图 1–117　髋关节（后面观）
Hip joint. Posterior aspect

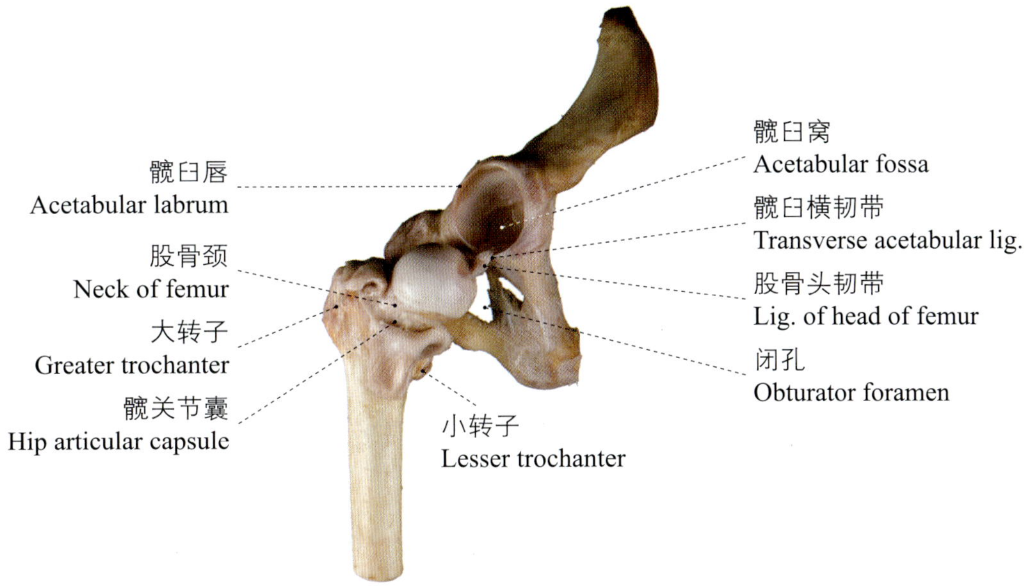

图 1–118　髋关节（打开关节囊）

Hip joint. Opened articular capsule

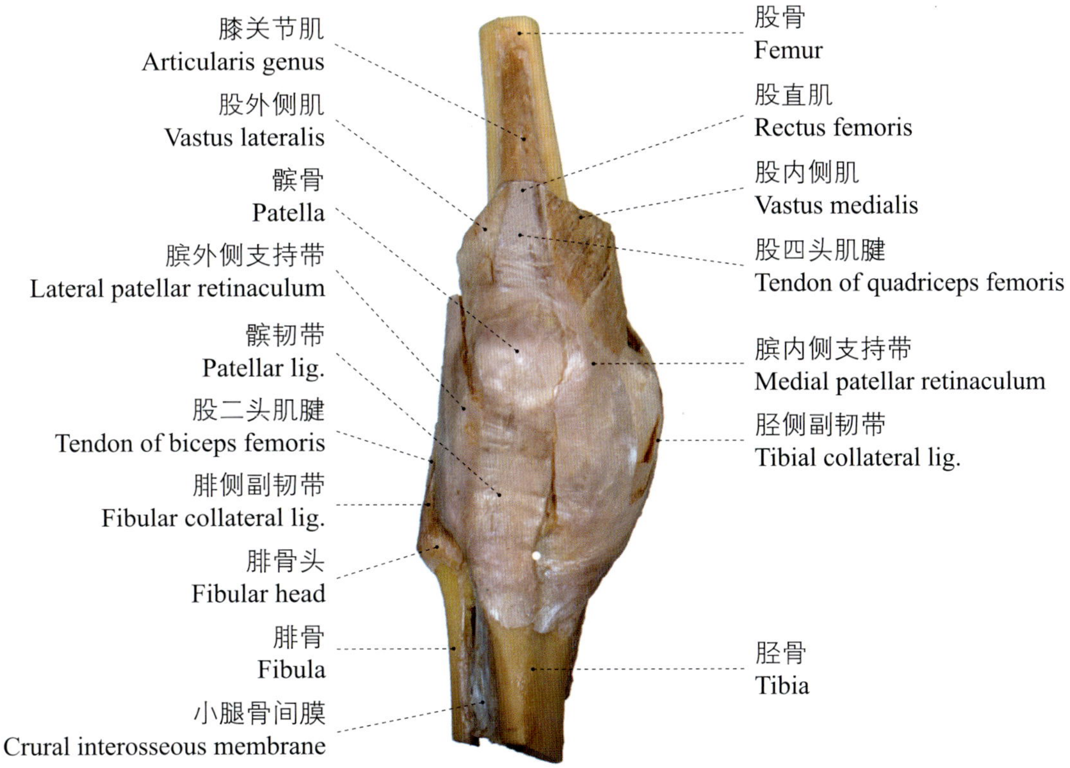

图 1–119　膝关节（前面观）

Knee joint. Anterior aspect

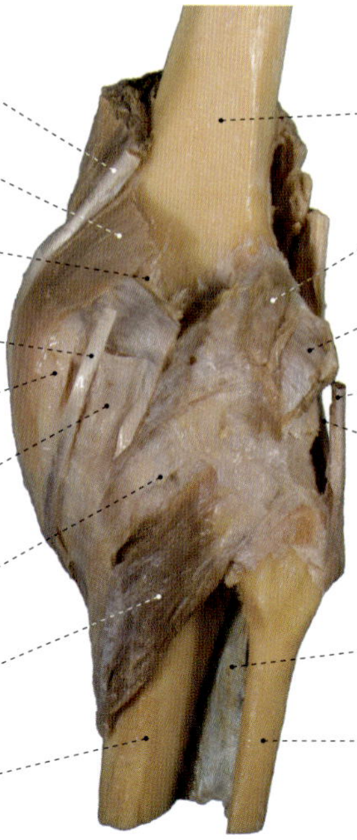

图 1–120　膝关节（后面观）

Knee joint. Posterior aspect

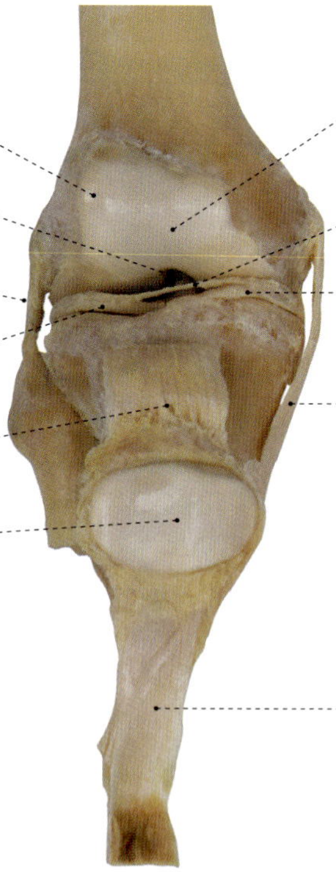

图 1–121　膝关节（前面观，打开关节囊）

Knee joint. Anterior aspect, opened articular capsule

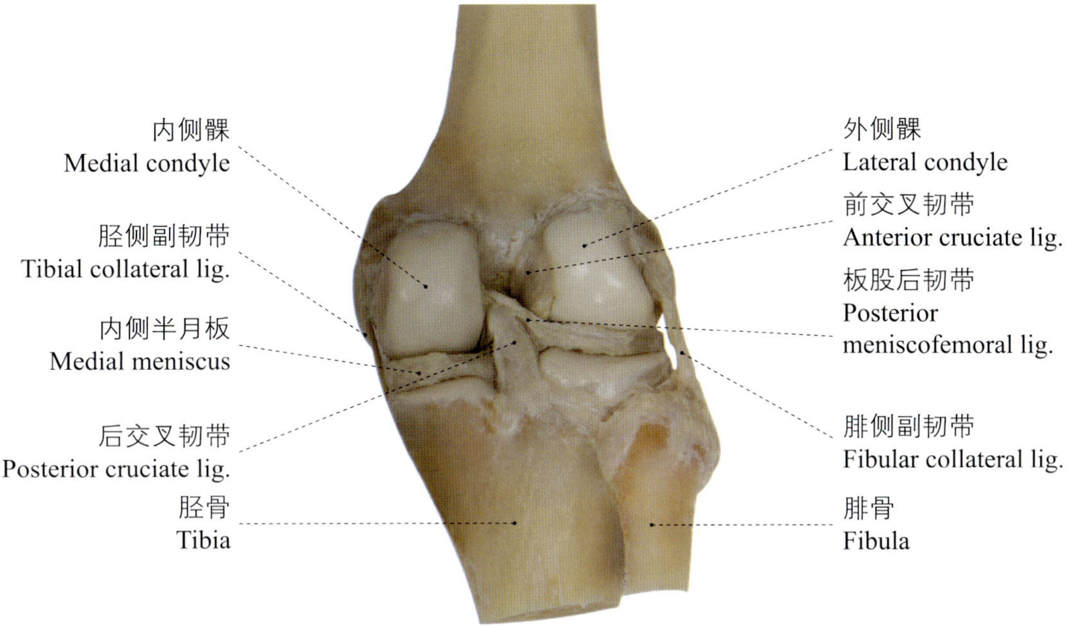

图 1–122　膝关节（后面观，打开关节囊）
Knee joint. Posterior aspect, opened articular capsule

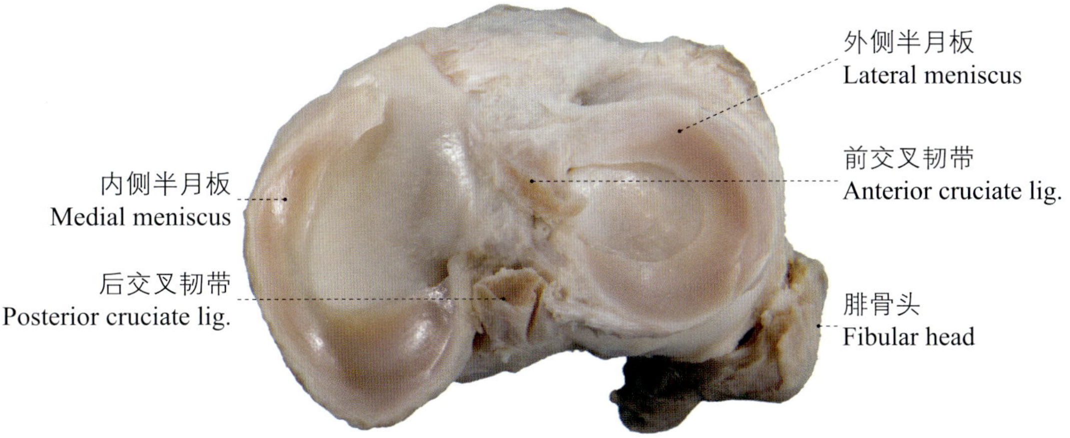

图 1–123　膝关节（上面观）
Knee joint. Superior aspect

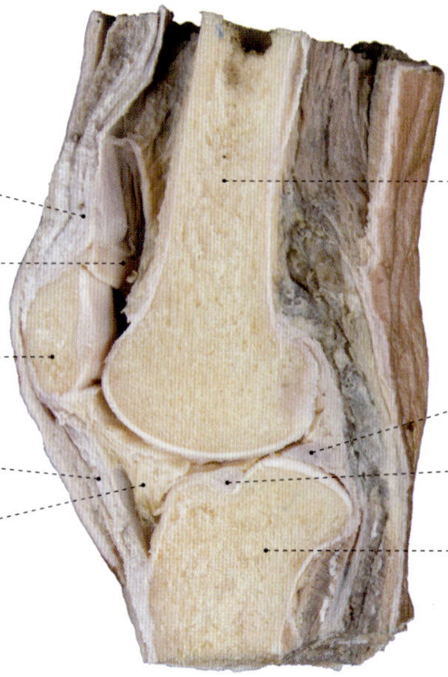

图 1–124　膝关节（矢状切面）

Knee joint. Sagittal aspect

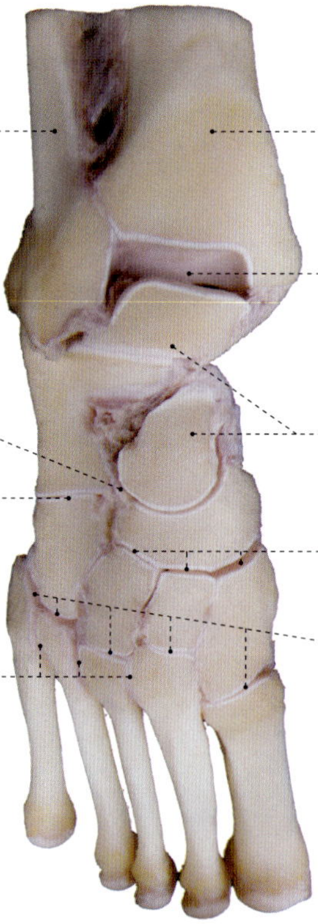

图 1–125　足的连结（水平和冠状切面）

Articulation of foot. Horizontal and coronal section

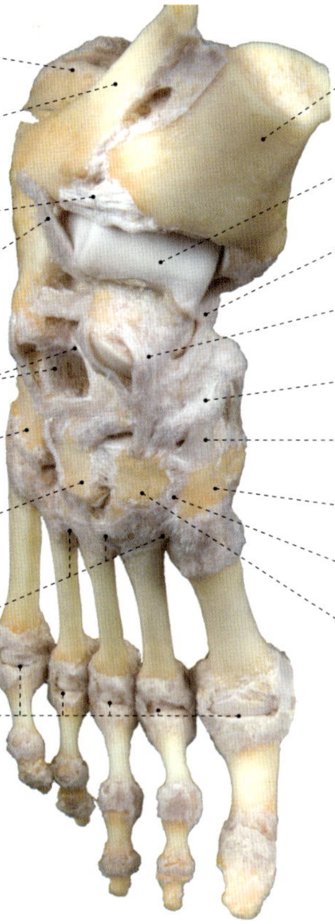

图 1–126　足的连结（上面观）

Articulation of foot. Superior aspect

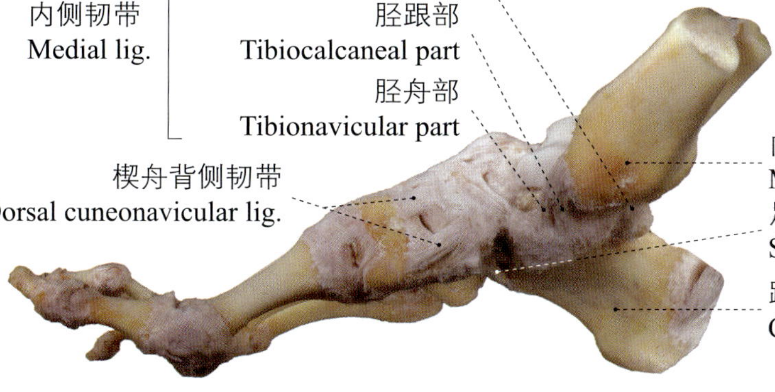

图 1–127　足的连结（内侧面观）

Articulation of foot. Medial aspect

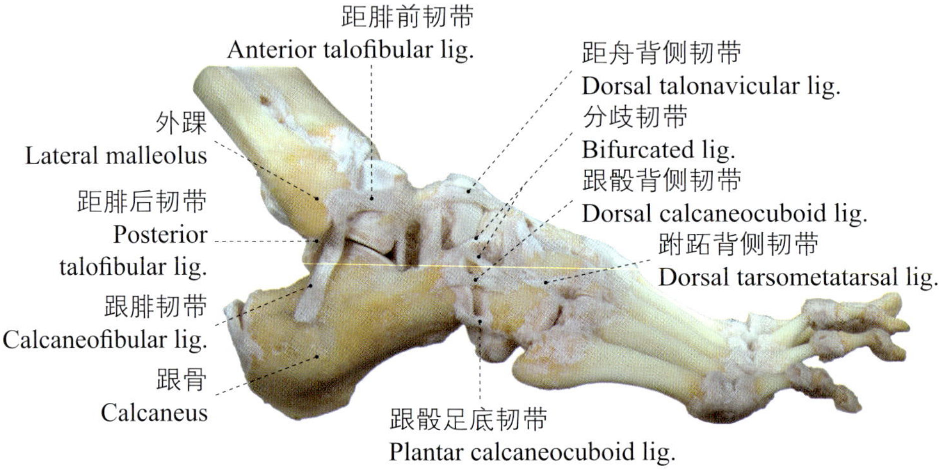

图 1–128　足的连结（外侧面观）

Articulation of foot. Lateral aspect

第三节　骨骼肌

头颈躯干肌

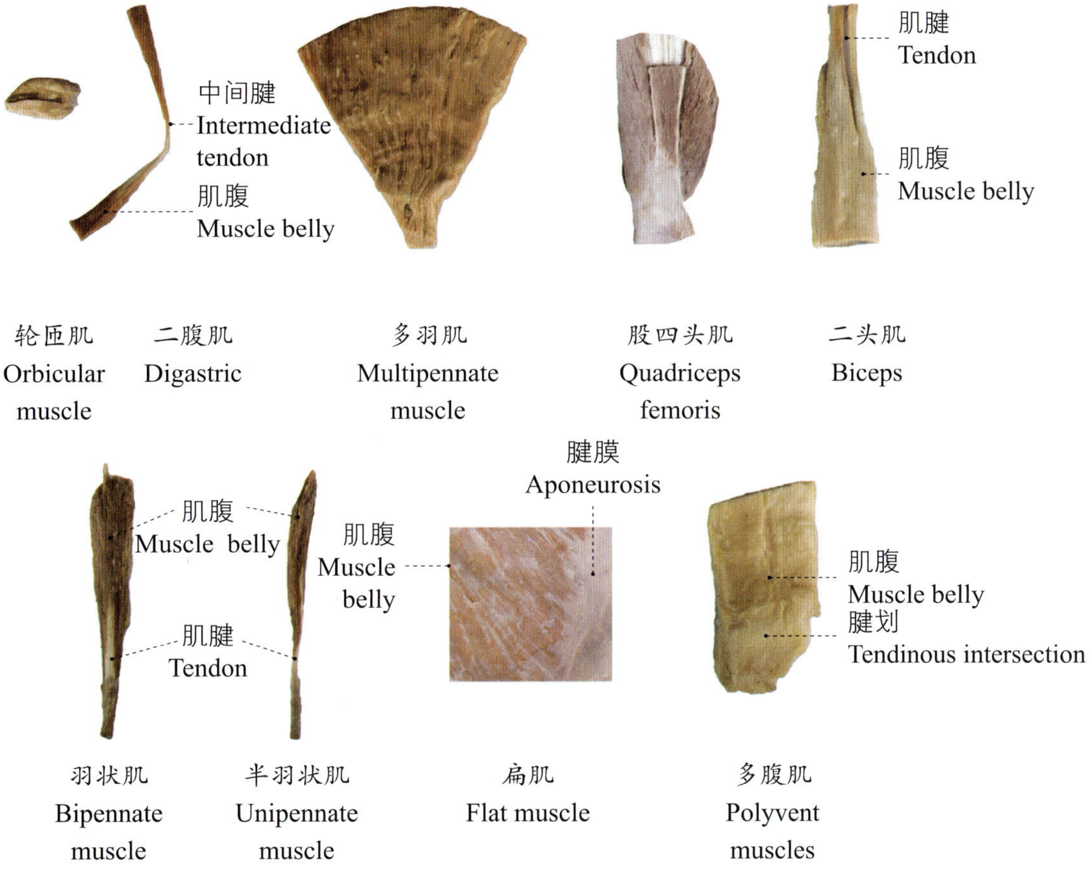

图 1–129　肌的形状

Forms of muscles

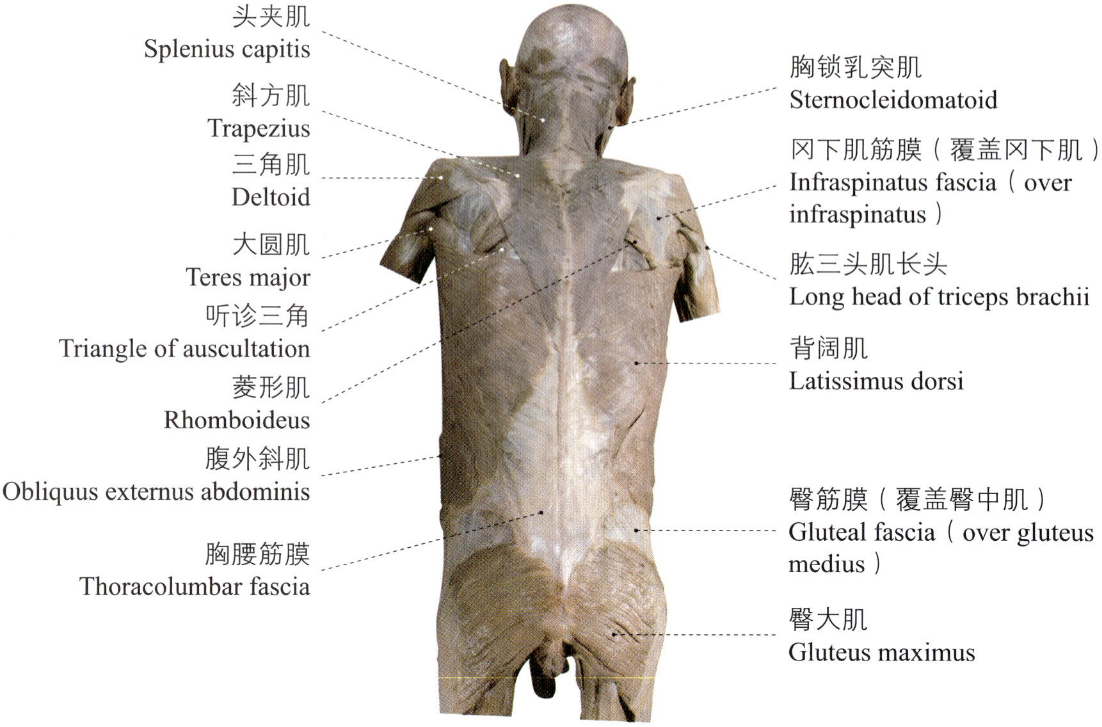

图 1–130　背部肌（1）

Muscles of back (1)

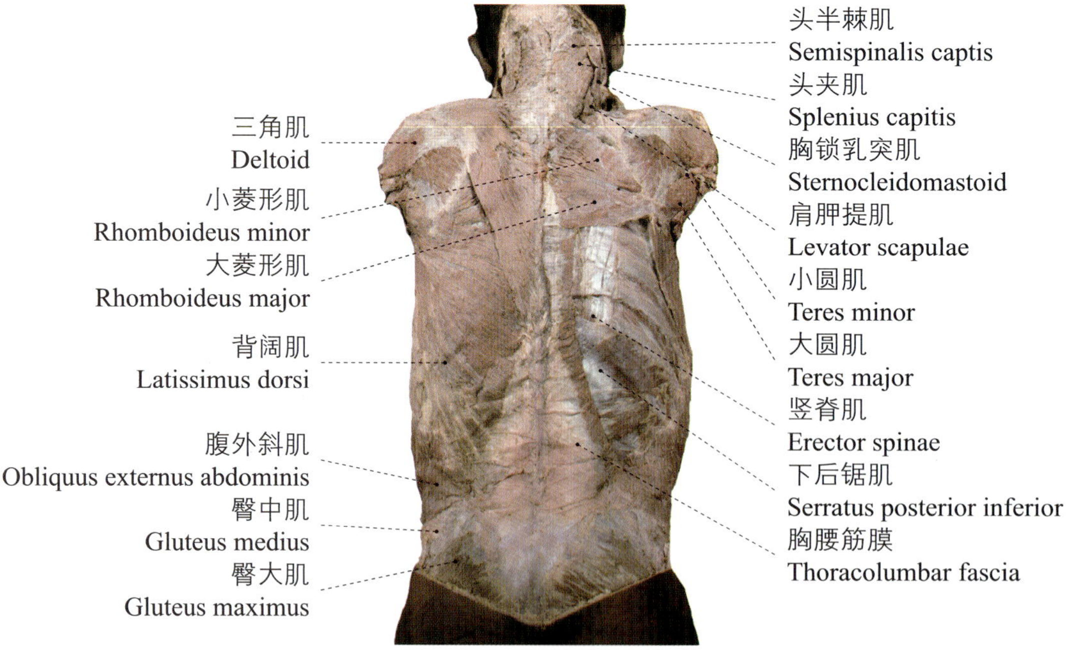

图 1–131　背部肌（2）

Muscles of back (2)

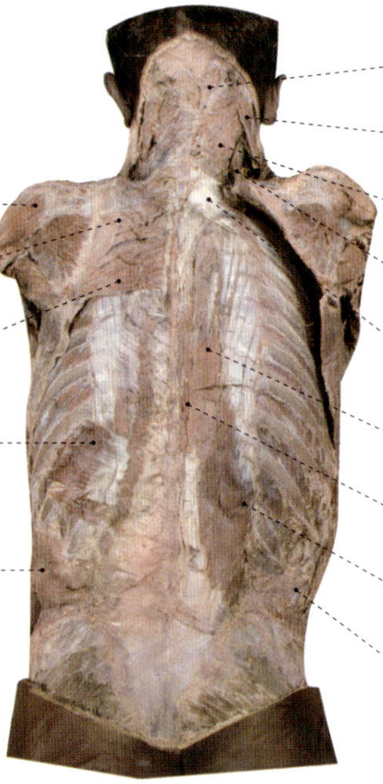

图 1–132　背部肌（3）
Muscles of back (3)

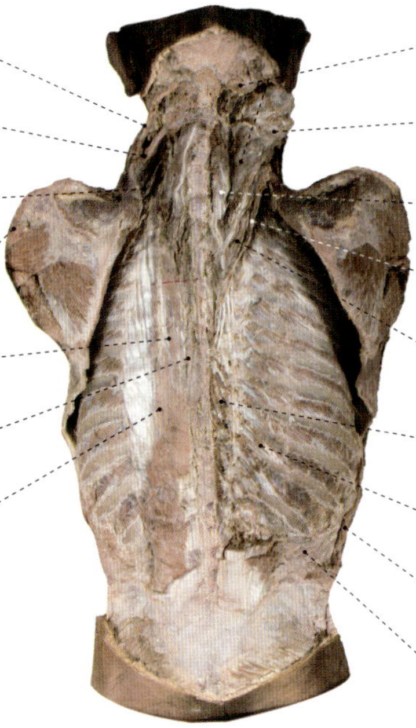

图 1–133　背部肌（4）
Muscles of back (4)

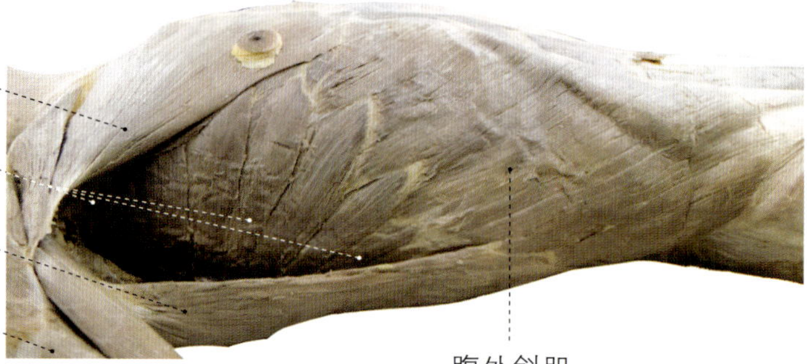

图 1–138　前锯肌（外侧面观）
Serratus anterior. Lateral aspect

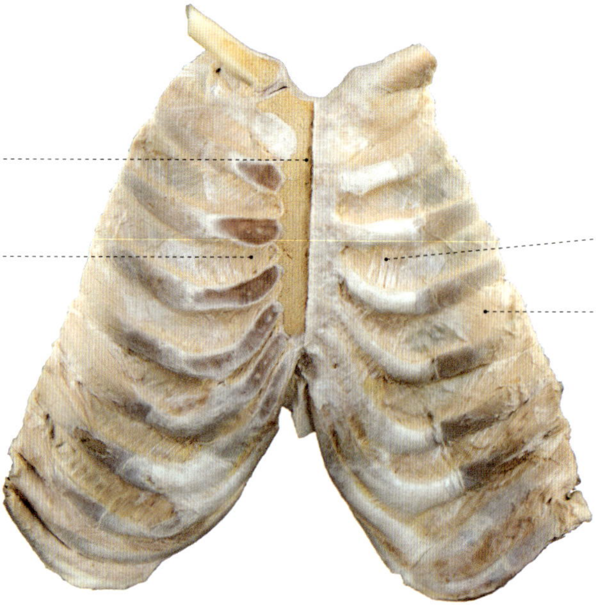

图 1–139　肋间肌
Intercostales

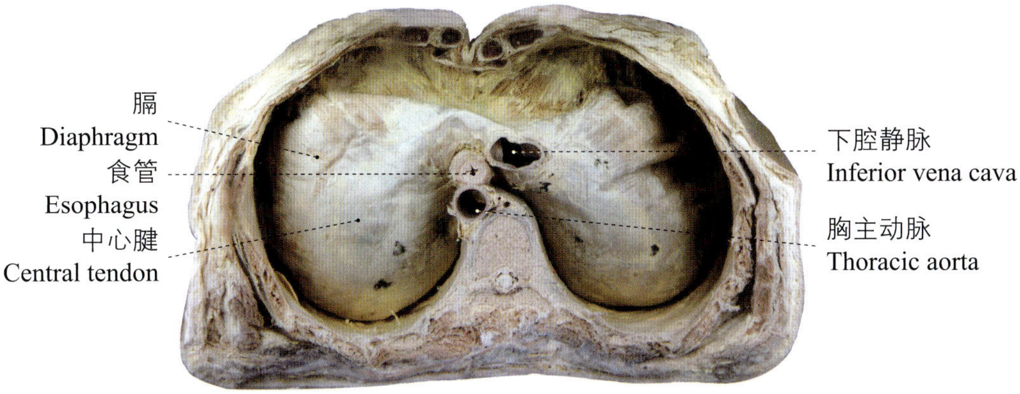

图 1–140 膈（上面观）
Diaphragm. Superior aspect

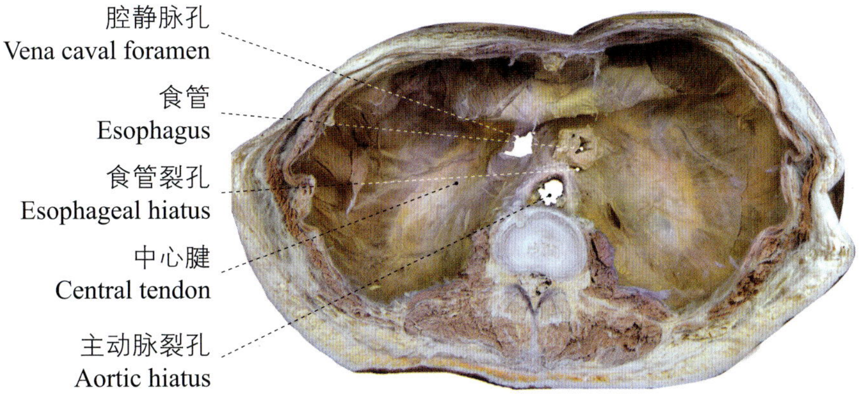

图 1–141 膈（下面观）
Diaphragm. Inferior aspect

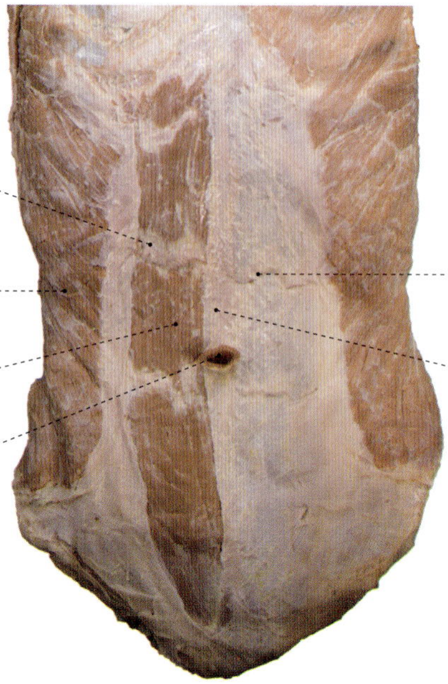

图 1–142 腹前外侧壁肌层（1）
Muscles layer of anterolateral abdominal wall (1)

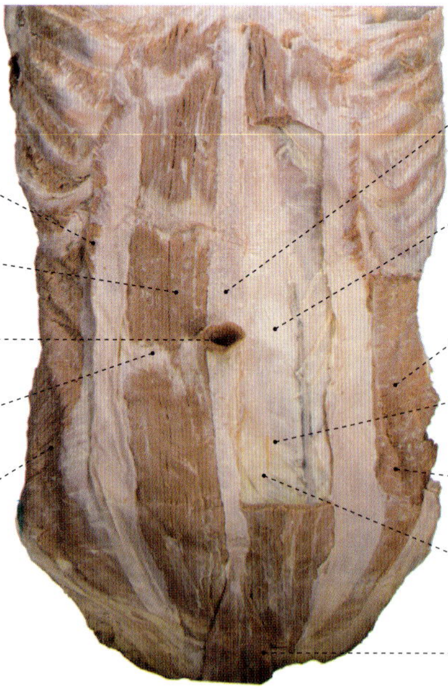

图 1–143 腹前外侧壁肌层（2）
Muscles layer of anterolateral abdominal wall (2)

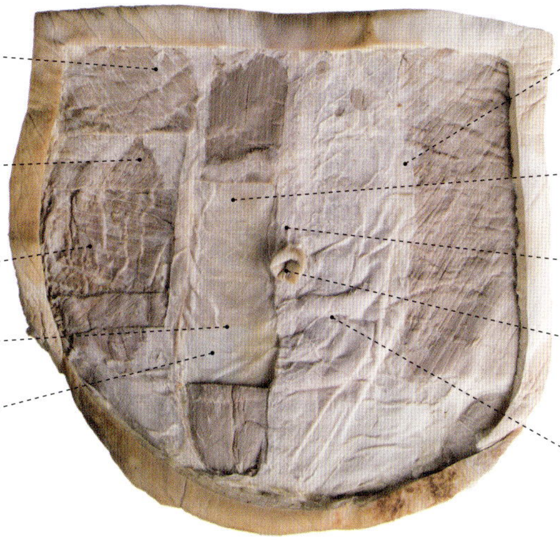

图 1–144　腹前外侧壁肌层（3）

Muscles layer of anterolateral abdominal wall (3)

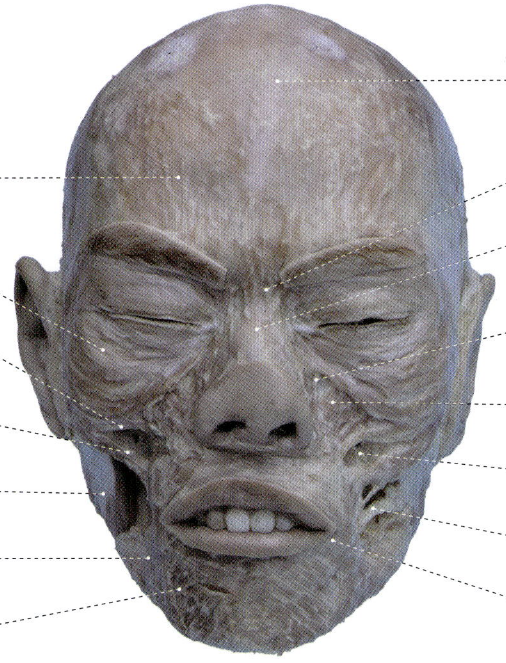

图 1–145　面部表情肌（前面观）

Muscles of facial expression. Anterior aspect

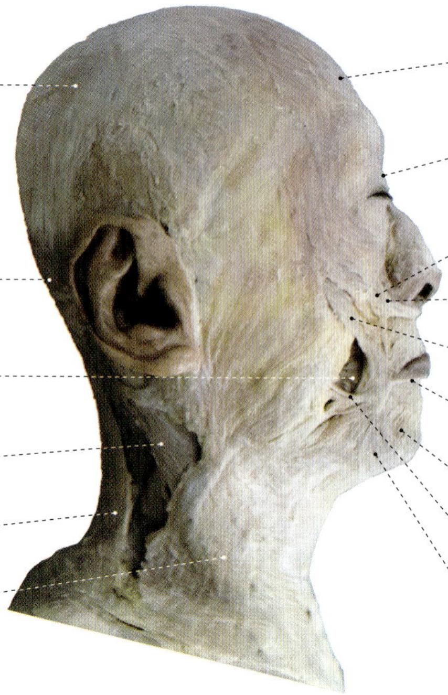

图 1–146　面部表情肌（侧面观）

Muscles of facial expression. Lateral aspect

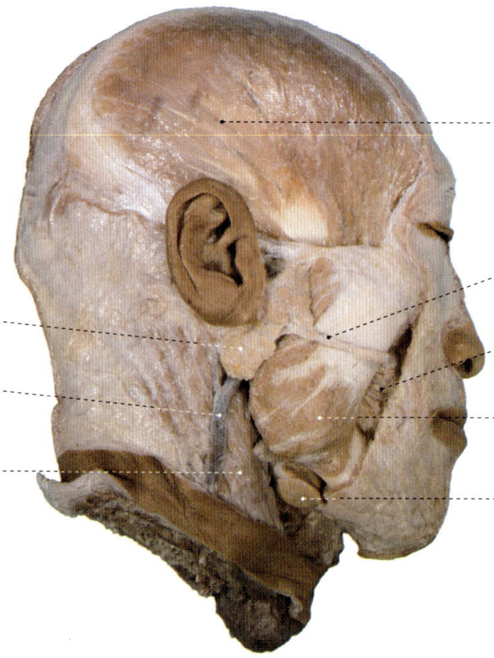

图 1–147　头部的肌（1）

Muscles of head (1)

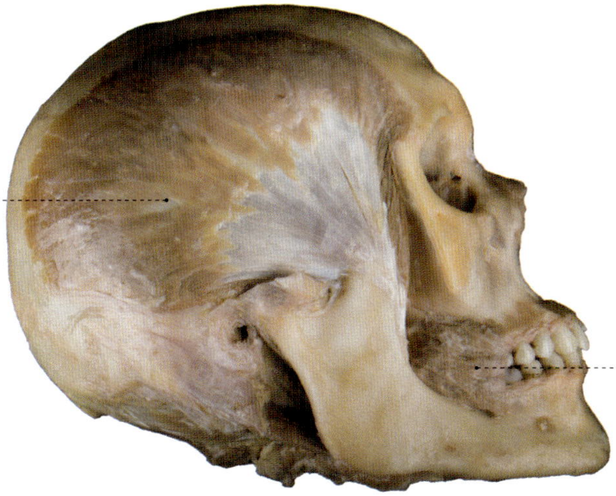

图 1–148　头部的肌（2）

Muscles of head (2)

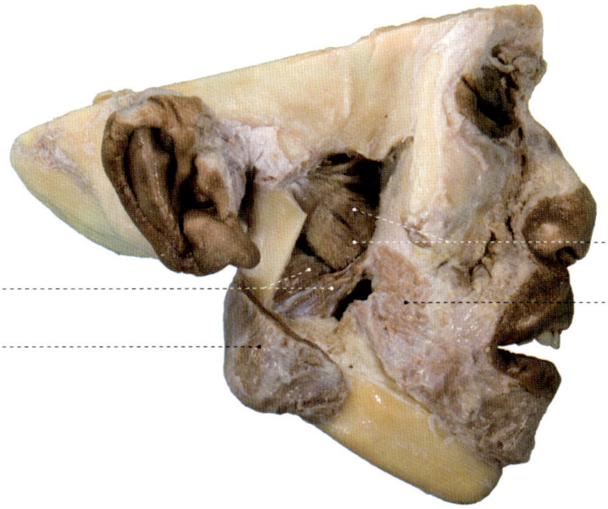

图 1–149　翼肌（外侧面观）

Pterygoid muscles. Lateral aspect

上肢肌

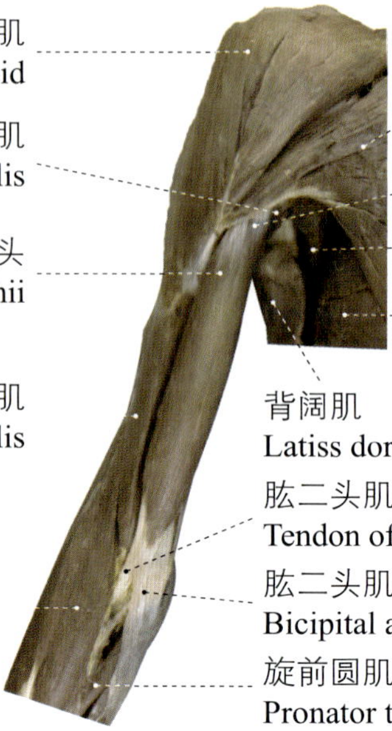

图 1–154　肩及臂部的肌肉（前面观）（1）

Muscles of shouder and arm. Anterior aspect (1)

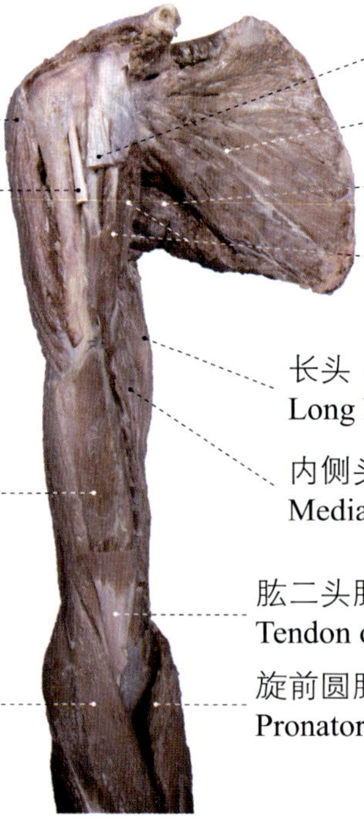

图 1–155　肩及臂部的肌肉（前面观）（2）

Muscles of shouder and arm. Anterior aspect (2)

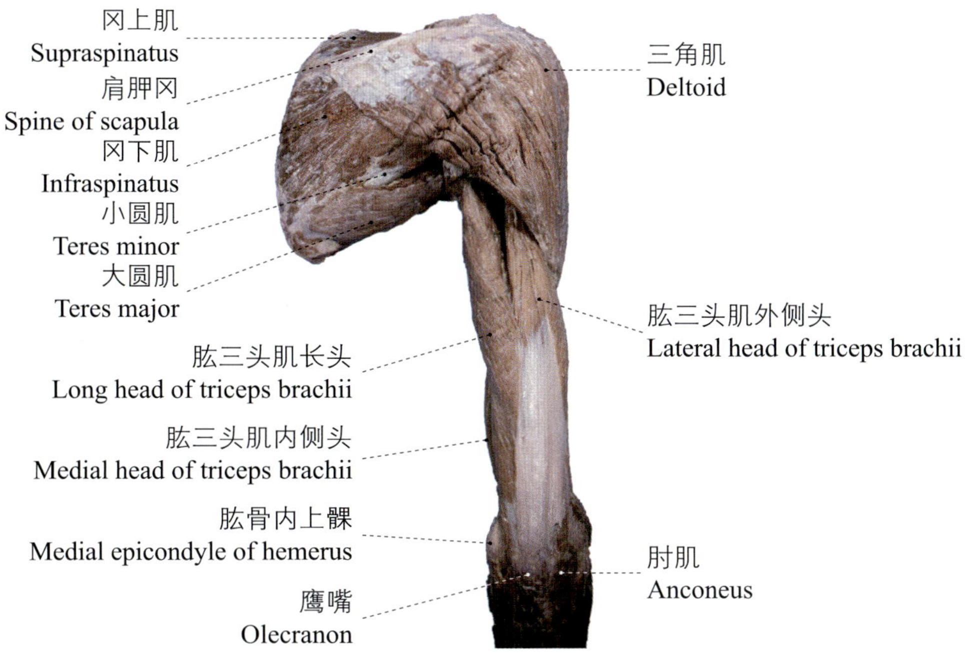

图 1–156　肩及臂部的肌肉（后面观）（1）

Muscles of shoulder and arm. Posterior aspect (1)

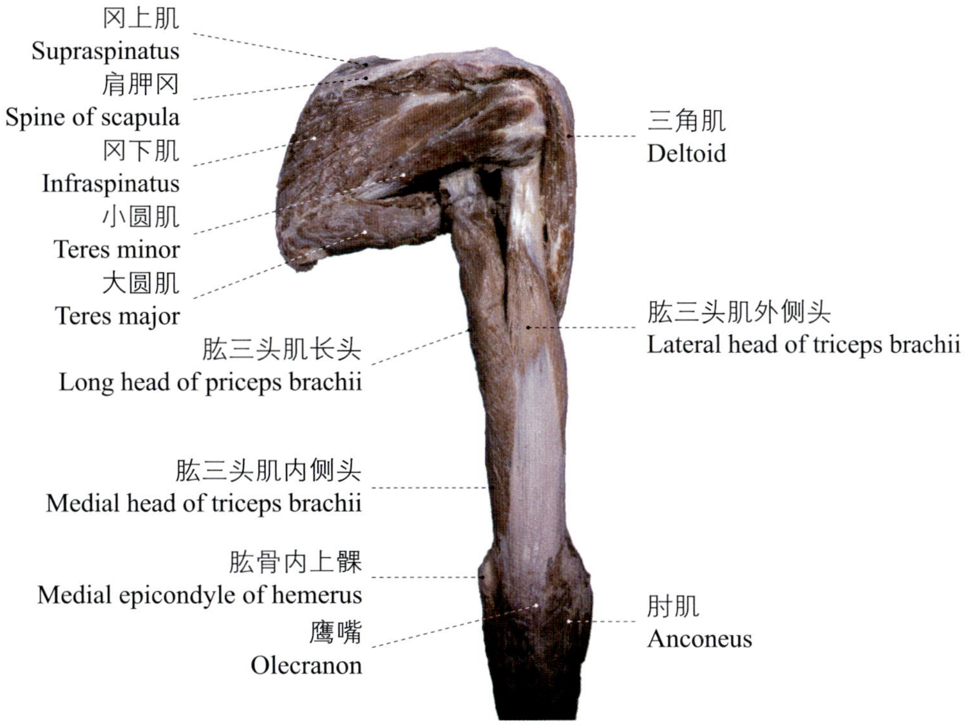

图 1–157　肩及臂部的肌肉（后面观）（2）

Muscles of shoulder and arm. Posterior aspect (2)

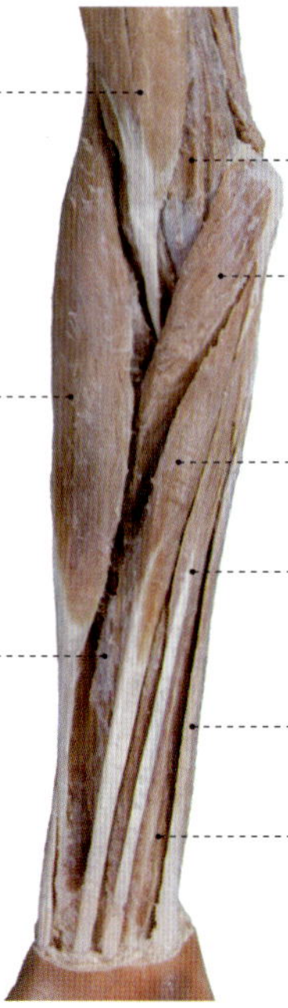

图 1–158 前臂肌（前面观）（1）

Muscles of forearm. Anterior aspect (1)

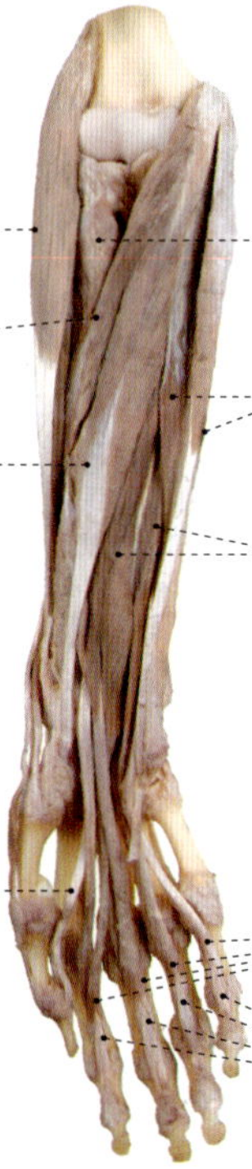

图 1–159 前臂肌（前面观）（2）

Muscles of forearm. Anterior aspect (2)

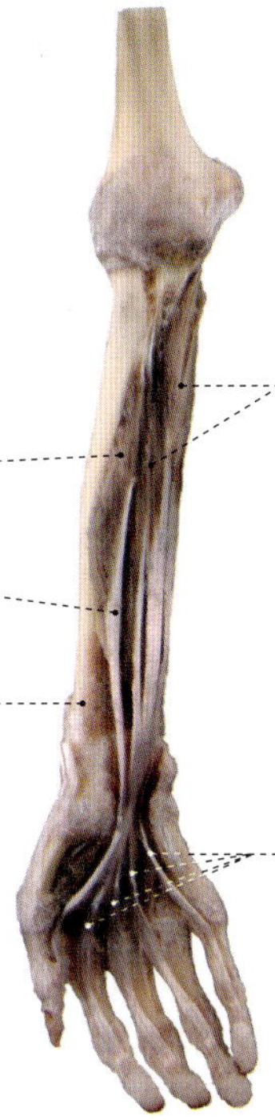

图 1-160　前臂肌（前面观）（3）

Muscles of forearm. Anterior aspect (3)

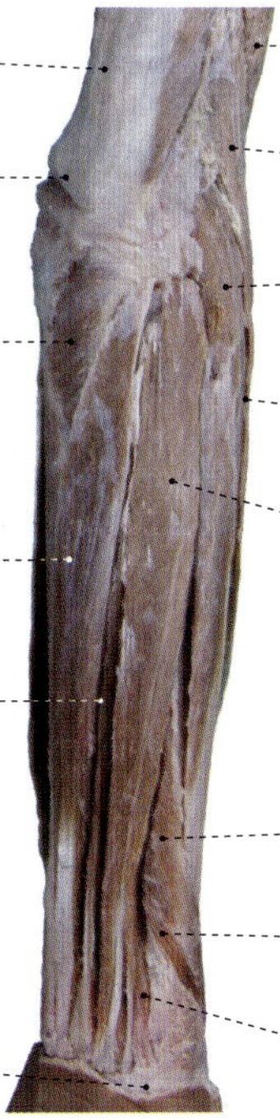

图 1-161　前臂肌（后面观）（1）

Muscles of forearm. Posterior aspect (1)

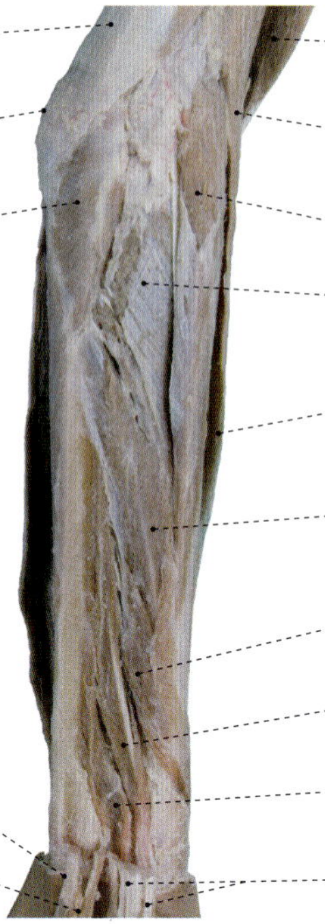

图 1–162　前臂肌（后面观）（2）

Muscles of forearm. Posterior aspect (2)

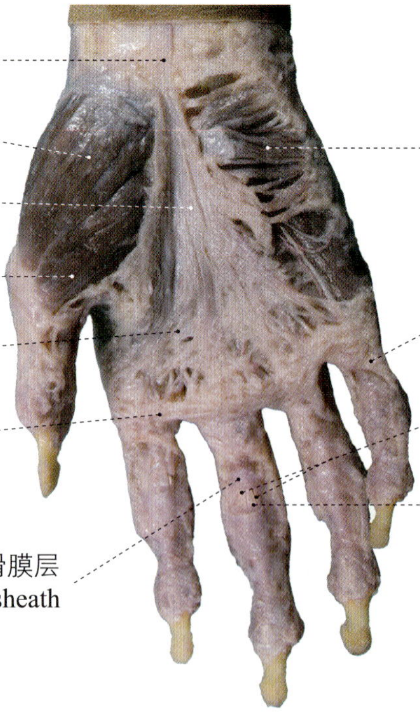

图 1–163　掌腱膜

Palmar aponeurosis

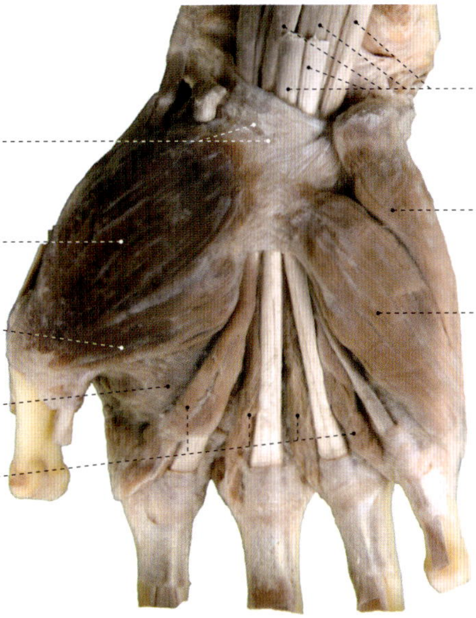

图 1–164 手肌（前面观）（1）
Muscles of hand. Anterior aspect (1)

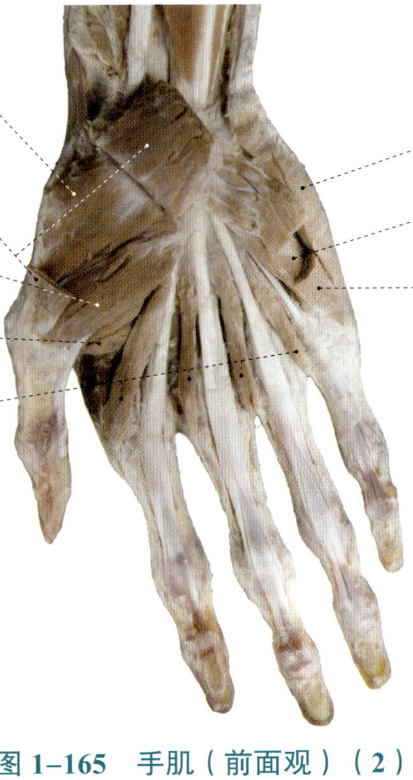

图 1–165 手肌（前面观）（2）
Muscles of hand. Anterior aspect (2)

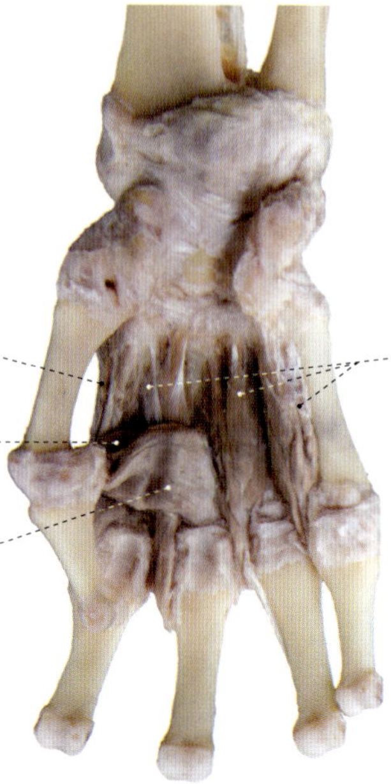

图 1-166　手肌（前面观）（3）

Muscles of hand. Anterior aspect (3)

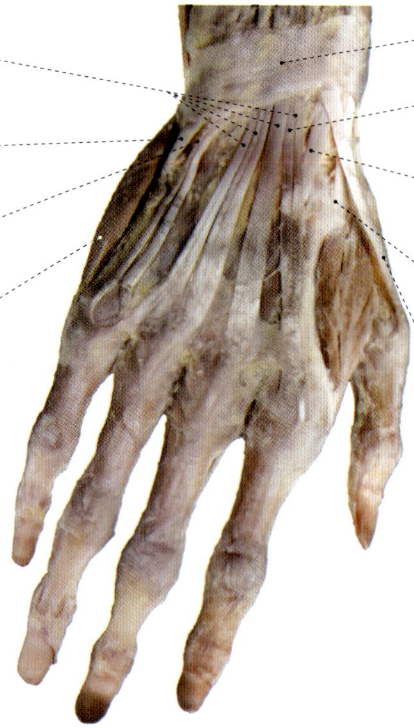

图 1-167　手背肌腱

Tendons of dorsum of hand

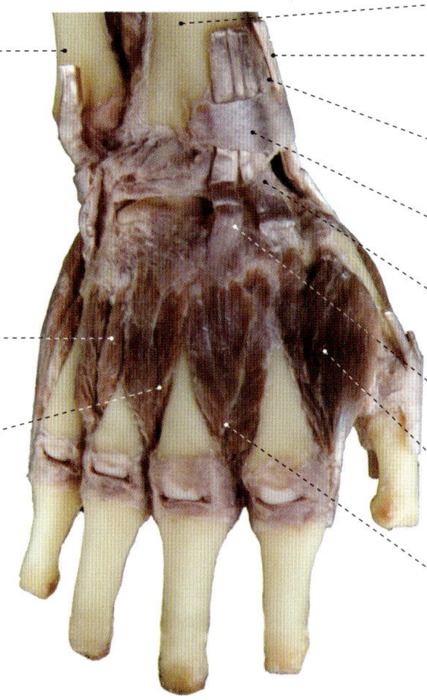

图 1–168　骨间背侧肌

Dorsal interossei

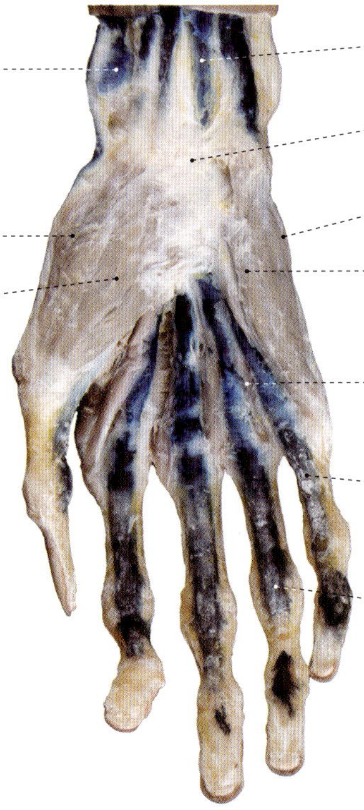

图 1–169　指腱鞘（前面观）

Tendnous sheaths of fingers. Anterior aspect

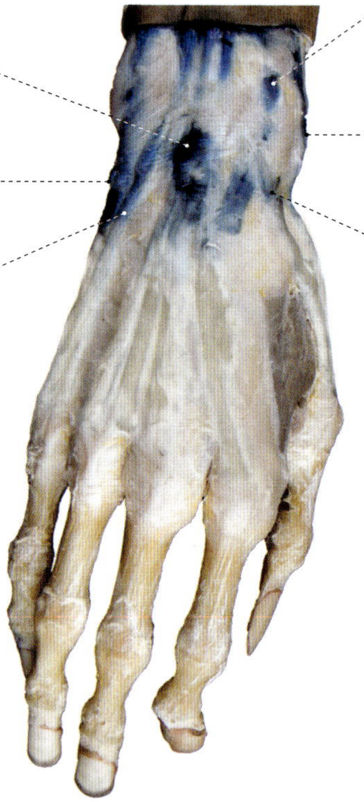

图 1–170　指腱鞘（后面观）

Tendinous sheaths of fingers. Posterior aspect

下肢肌

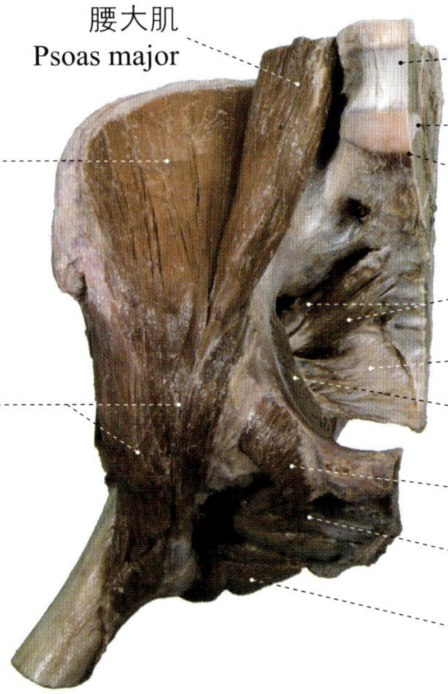

图 1–171　髋肌（前面观）
Muscles of hip. Anterior aspect

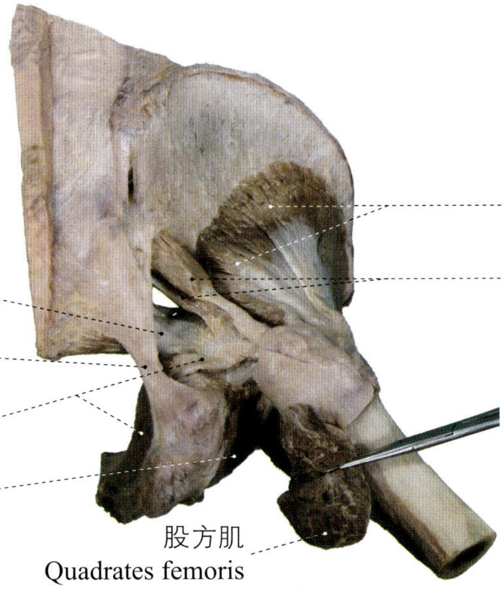

图 1–172　髋肌（后面观）
Muscles of hip. Posterior aspect

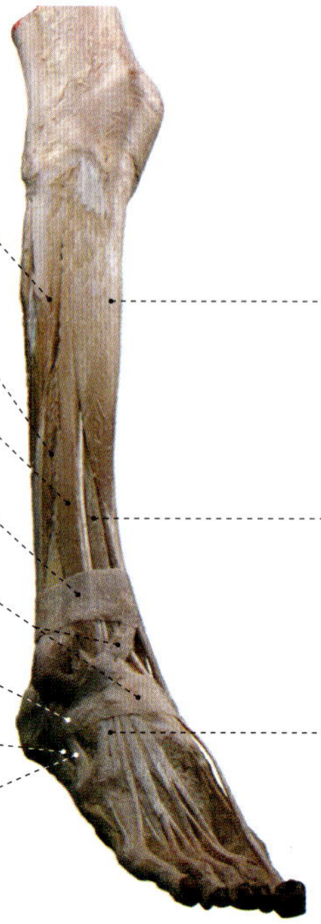

图 1–177　小腿肌（前外侧面观）

Muscles of leg. Anterolateral aspect

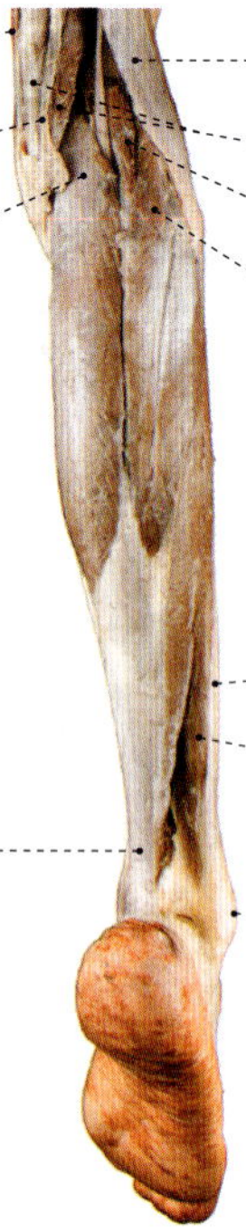

图 1–178　小腿肌（后面观）（1）

Muscles of leg. Posterior aspect (1)

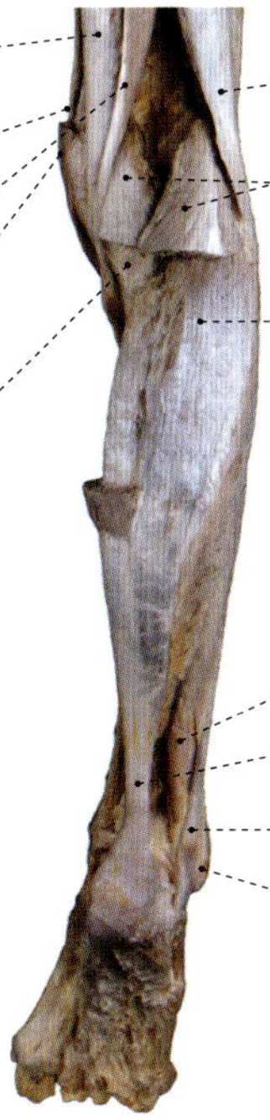

图 1–179 小腿肌（后面观）（2）
Muscles of leg. Posterior aspect (2)

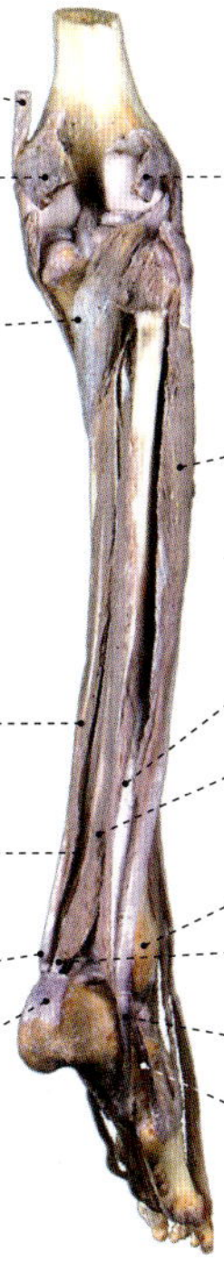

图 1–180 小腿肌（后面观）（3）
Muscles of leg. Posterior aspect (3)

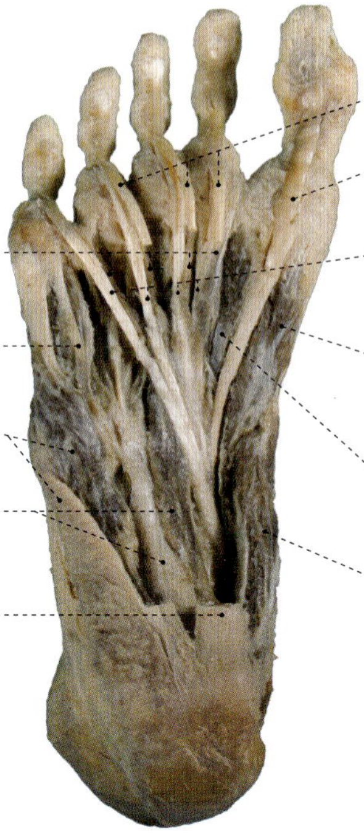

图 1–185 足底肌（3）

Muscles of sole of foot (3)

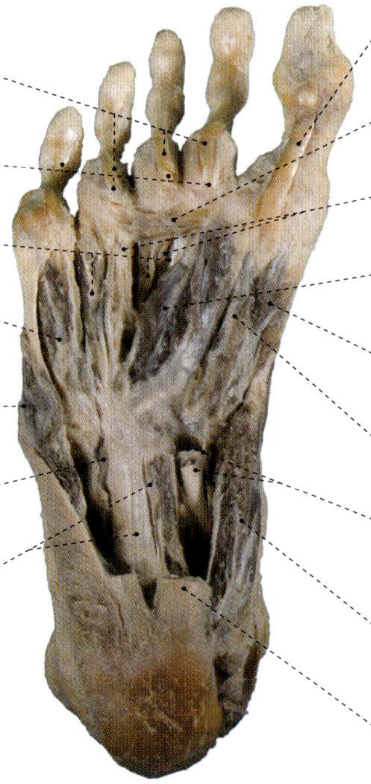

图 1–186 足底肌（4）

Muscles of sole of foot (4)

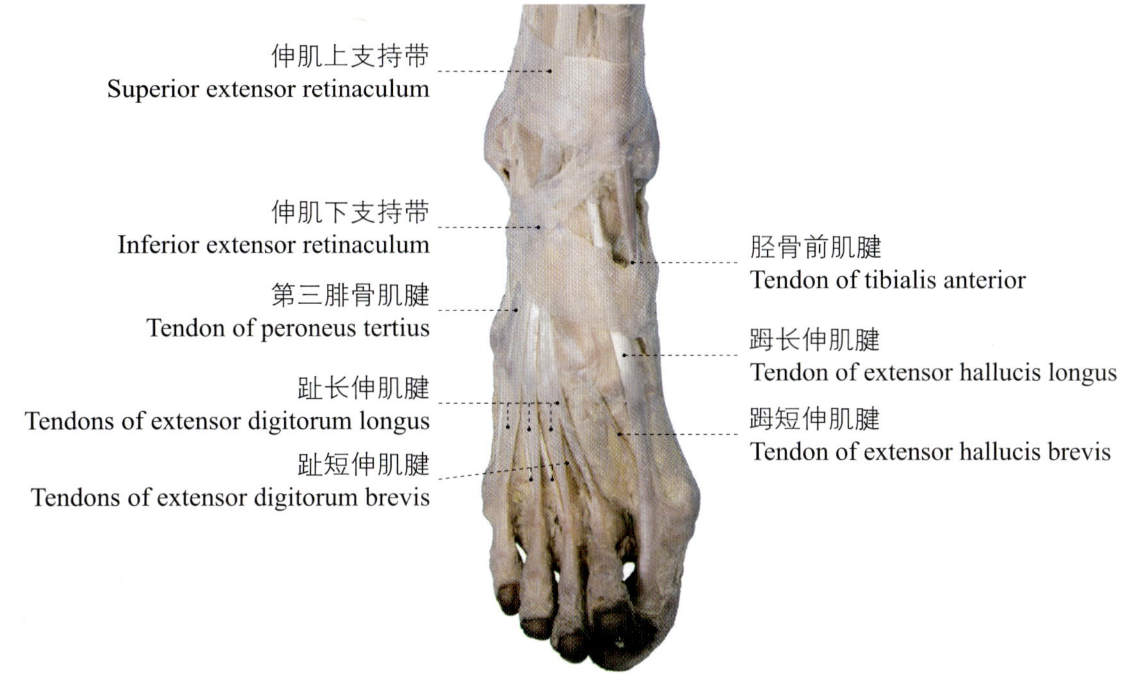

图 1–187　足肌（上面观）

Muscles of foot. Superior aspect

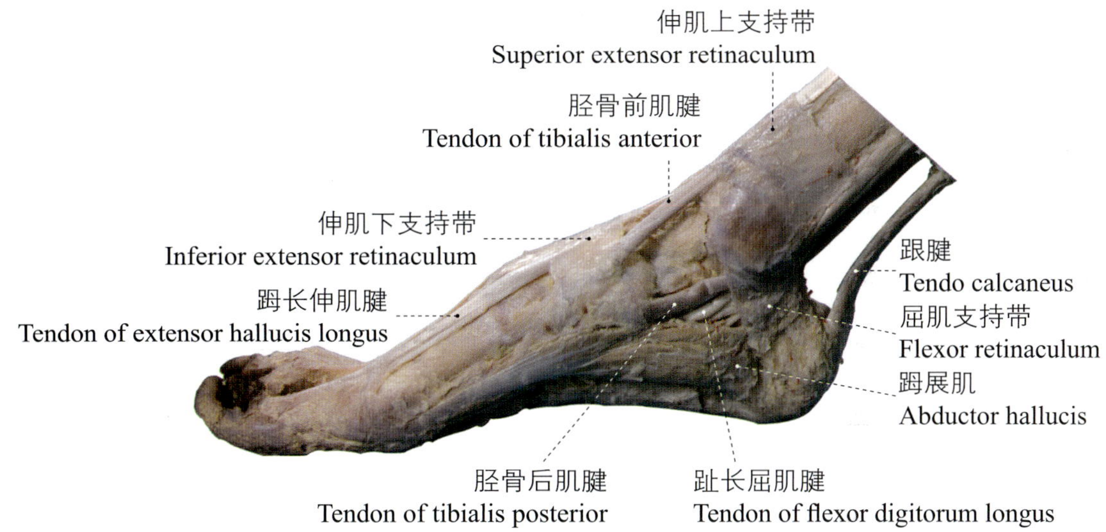

图 1–188　足肌（内侧面观）

Muscles of foot. Medial aspect

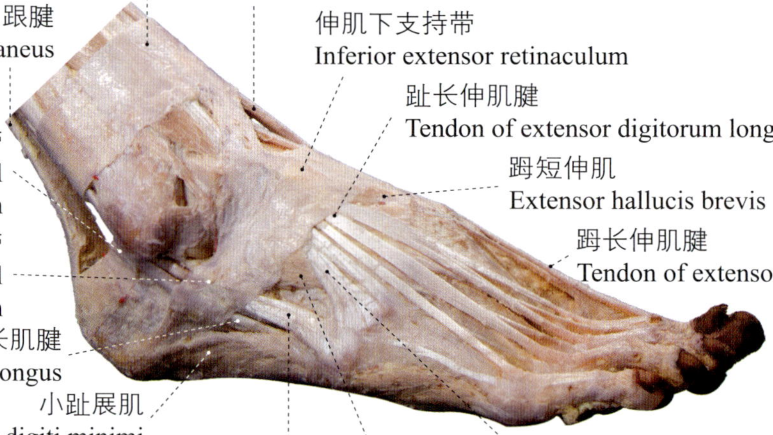

图 1–189　足肌（外侧面观）

Muscles of foot. Lateral aspect

第二章　消化系统

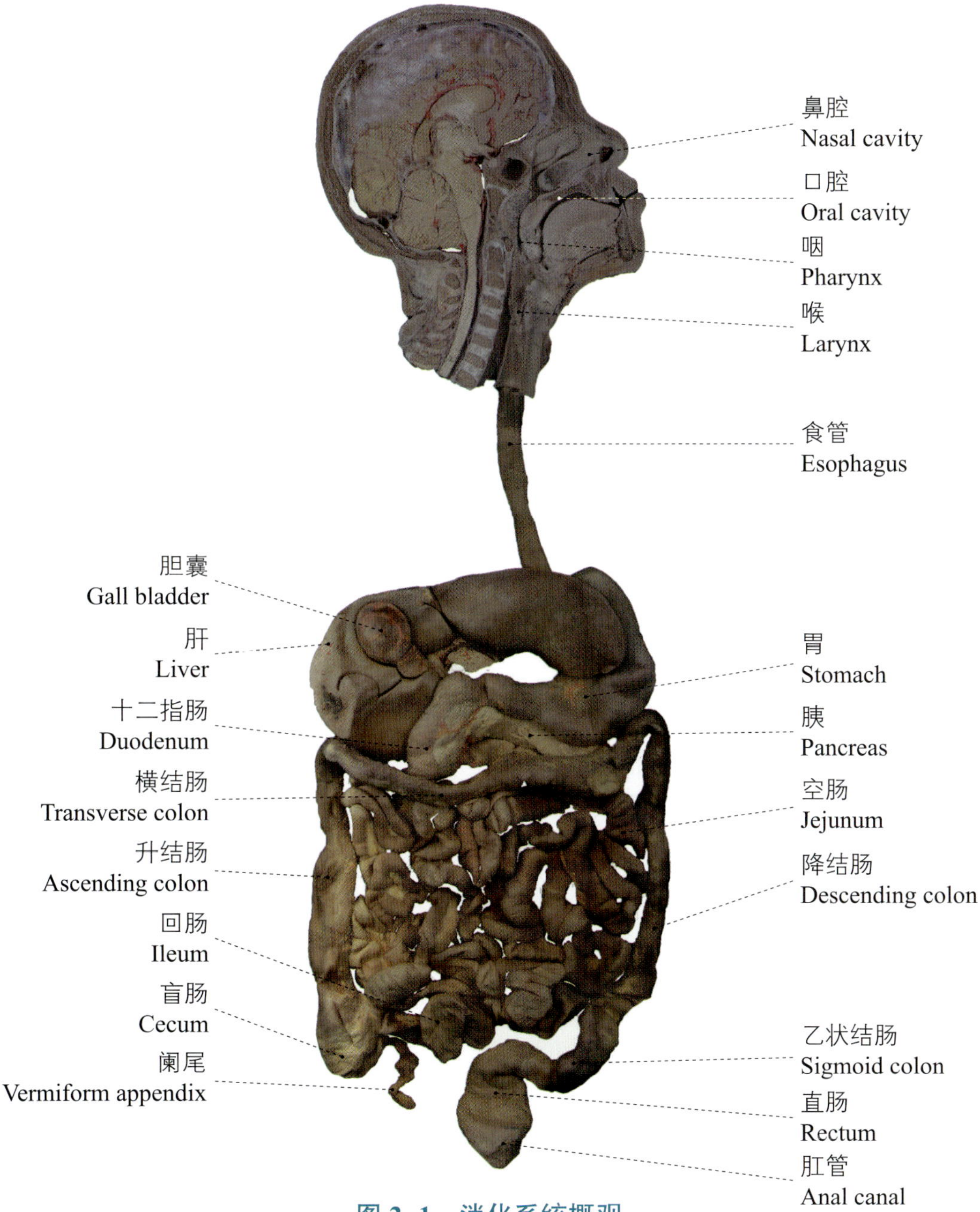

图 2–1　消化系统概观

Gerneral arrangement of digestive system

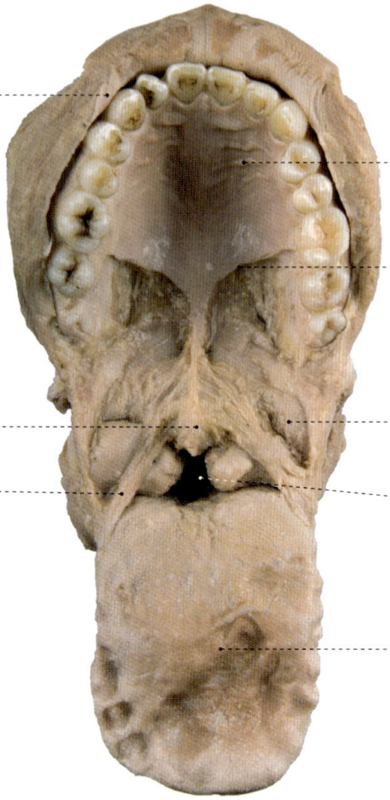

图 2–2 口腔和咽峡

Oral cavity and isthmus of fauces

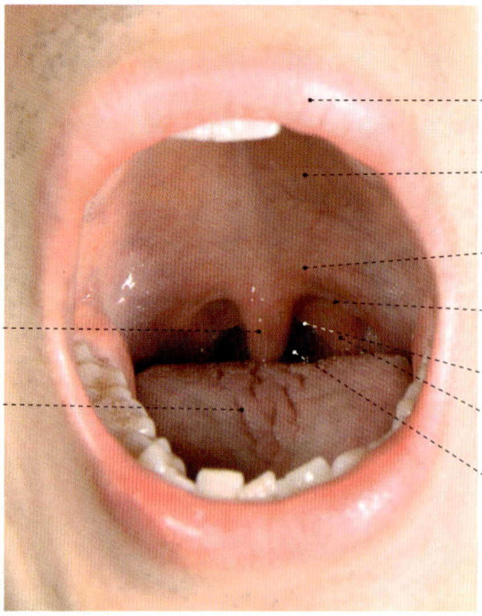

图 2–3 口腔（1）

Oral cavity (1)

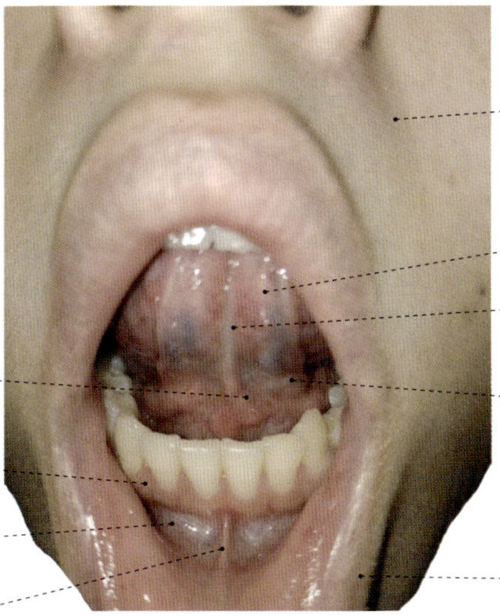

图 2-4　口腔（2）

Oral cavity (2)

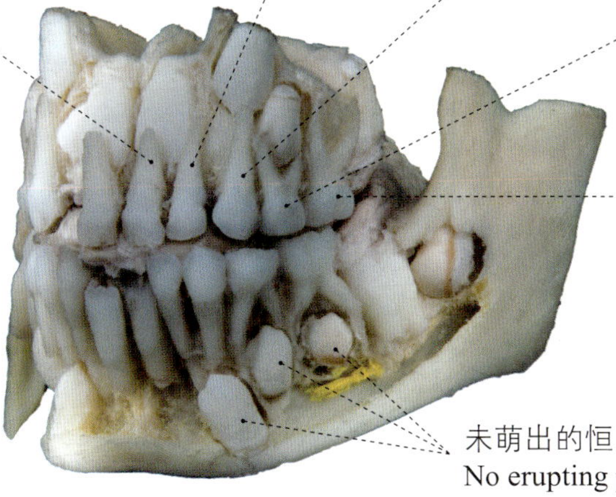

图 2-5　乳牙

Deciduous teeth

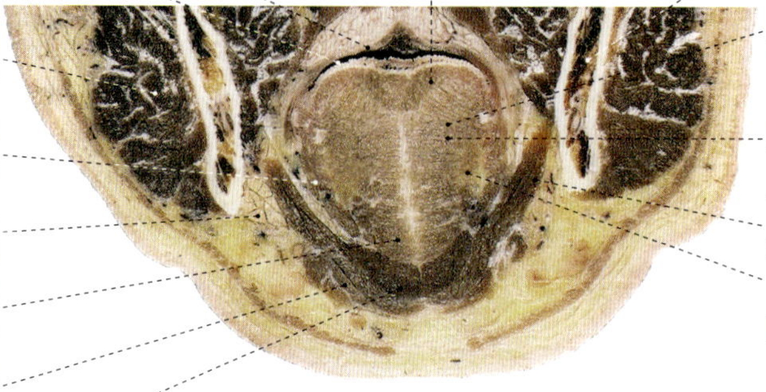

图 2-10　舌肌（冠状切面）
Muscles of tongue. Coronal section

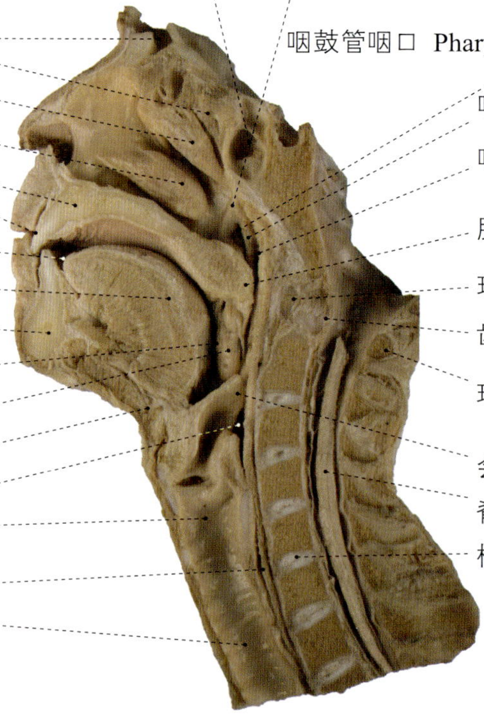

图 2-11　头颈部（正中矢状切面）
Head and neck. Median sagittal section

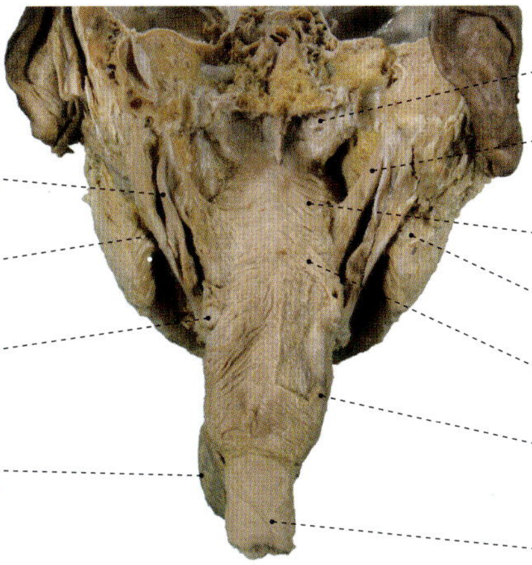

图 2-12　咽肌（后面观）

Muscles of pharynx. Posterior aspect

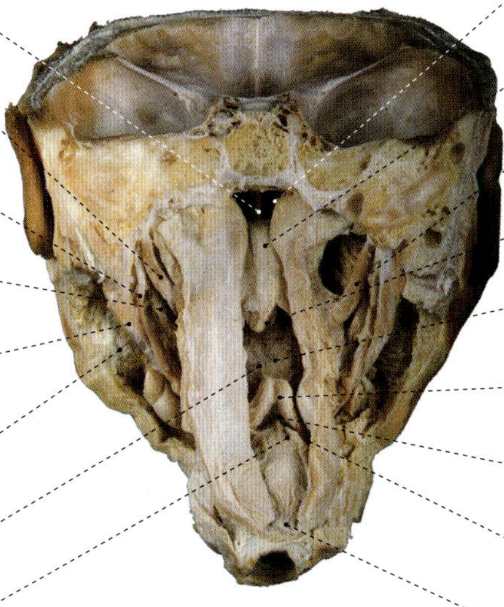

图 2-13　咽腔（后面观）

Pharyngeal cavity. Posterior aspect

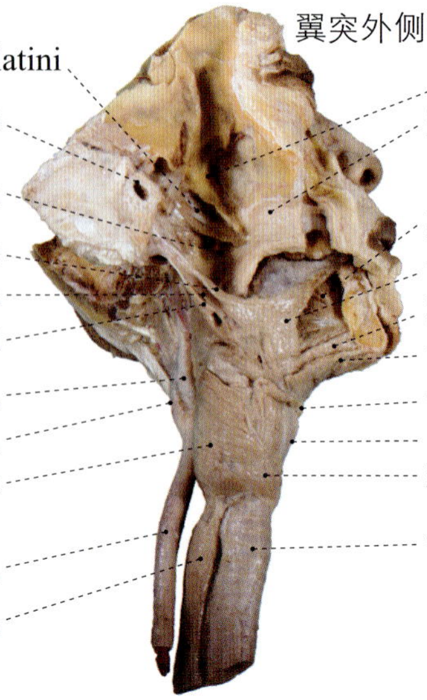

图 2-14　咽（外侧面观）

Pharynx Lateral aspect

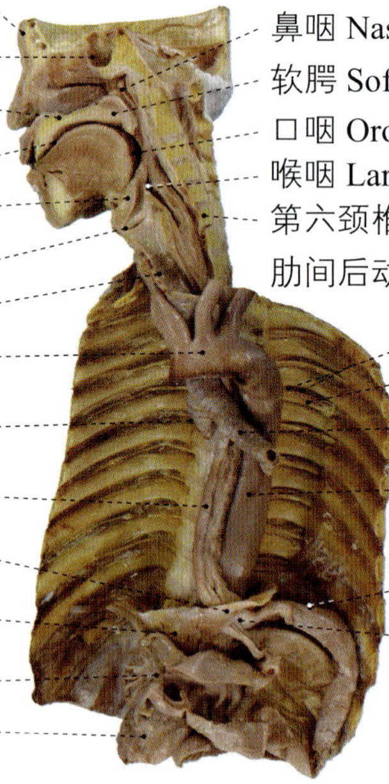

图 2-15　食管

Esophagus

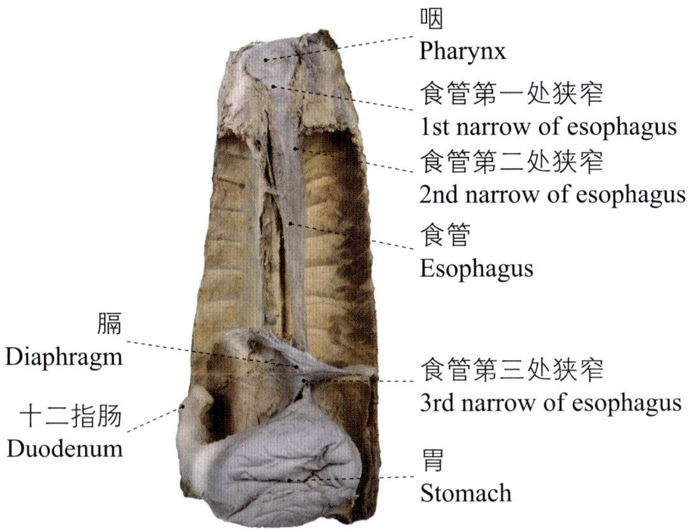

图 2–16　食管（前面观）

Esophagus. Anterior aspect

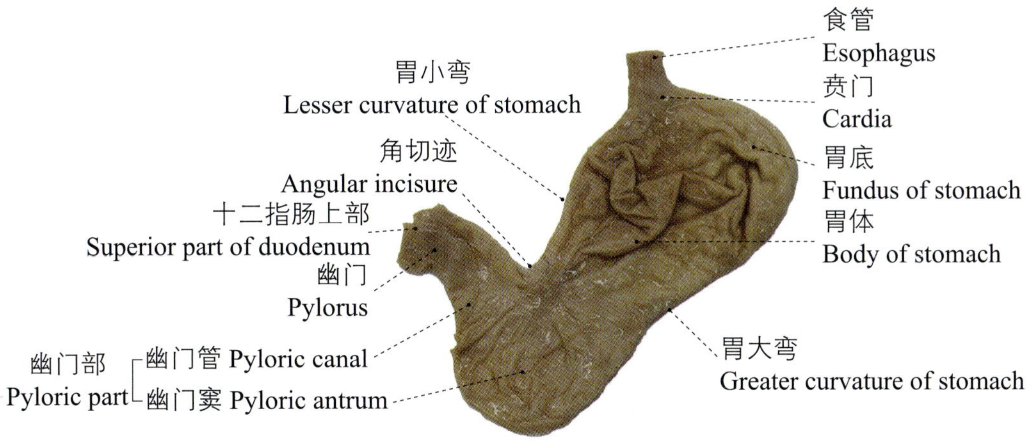

图 2–17　胃的形态和分部

Shape and subdivisions of stomach

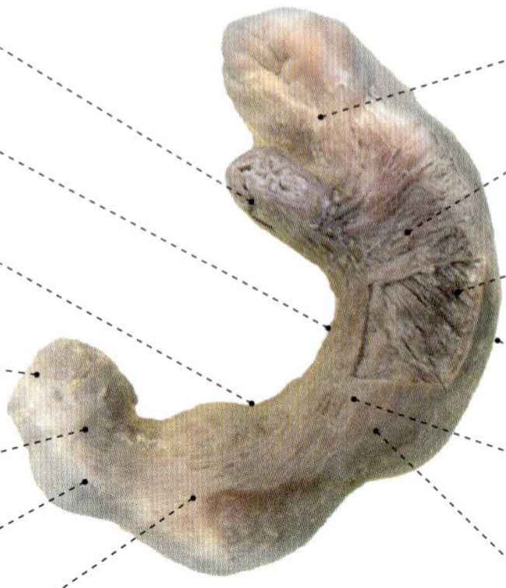

图 2-18　胃的肌层和分部

Muscular coat and subdivisions of stomach

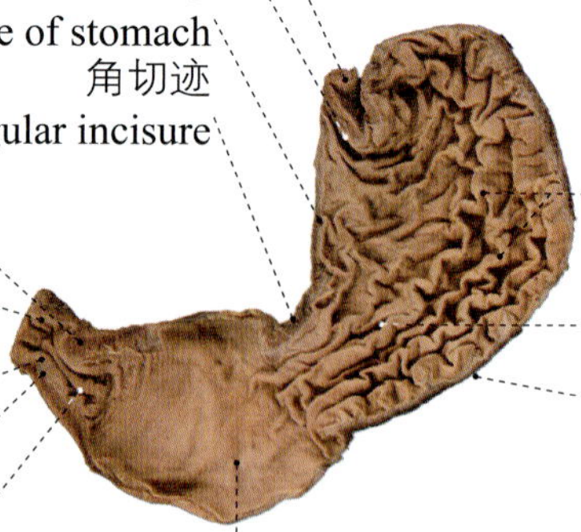

图 2-19　胃黏膜

Mucous membrane of stomach

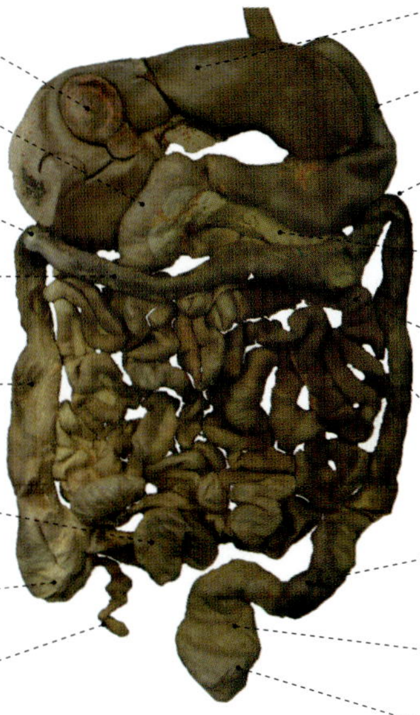

图 2–20　消化系统脏器（前面观）

Viscera of digestive system. Anterior aspect

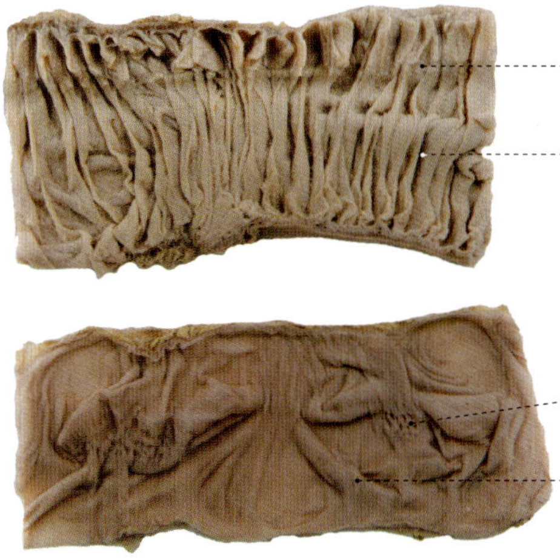

图 2–21　空肠和回肠的黏膜

Mucous membrane of jejunum and ileum

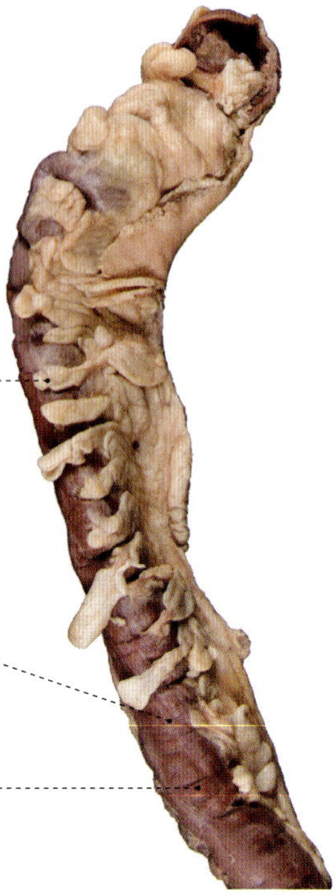

图 2–22　结肠（外面观）
Colon. External aspect

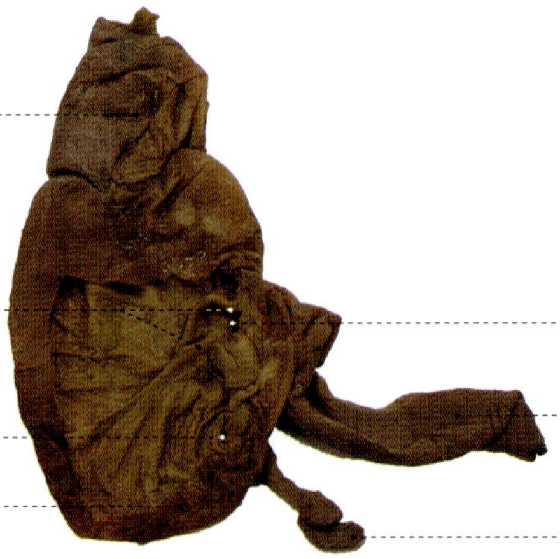

图 2–23　盲肠与阑尾
Cecum and vermiform appendix

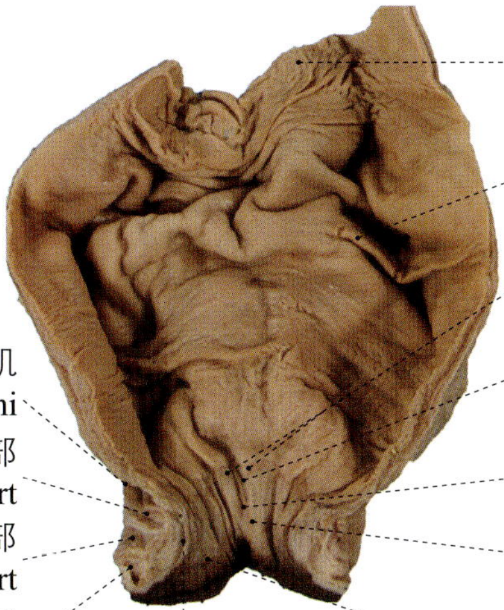

图 2–24　直肠与肛管（内面观）

Rectum and anal canal. Internal aspect

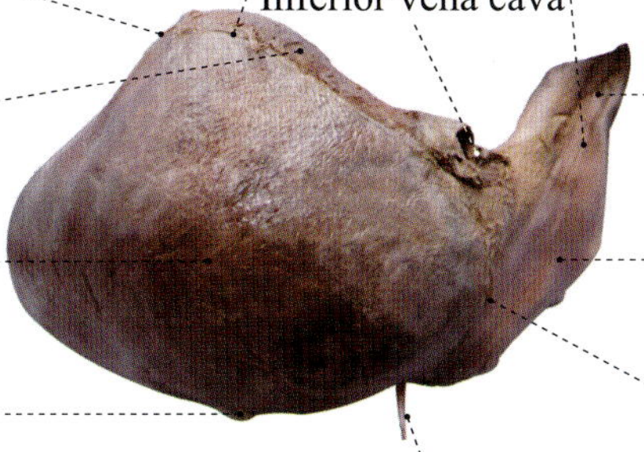

图 2–25　肝（上面观）

Liver. Superior aspect

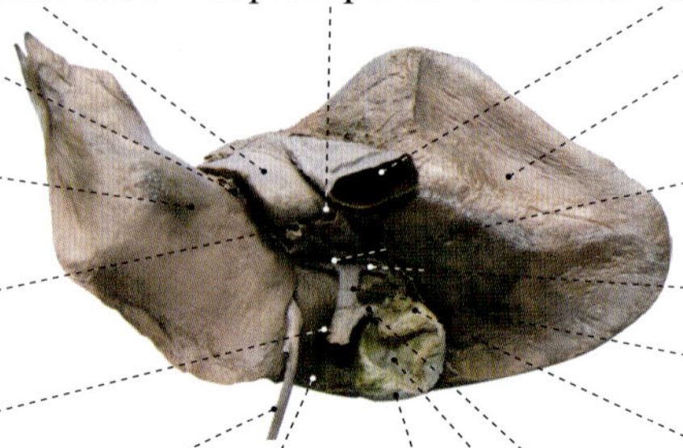

图 2-26　肝（下面观）

Liver. Inferior aspect

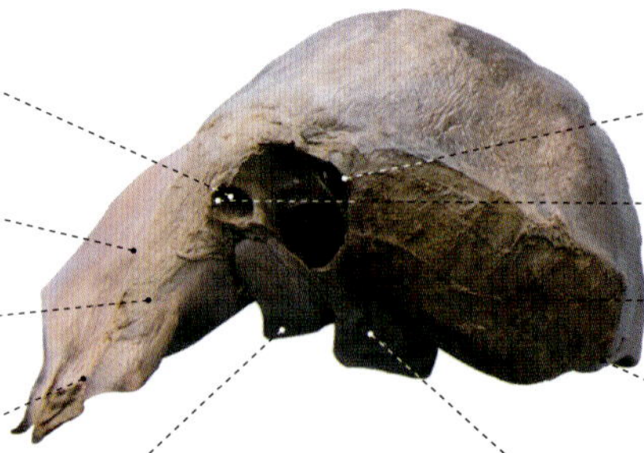

图 2-27　肝（后面观）

Liver. Posterior aspect

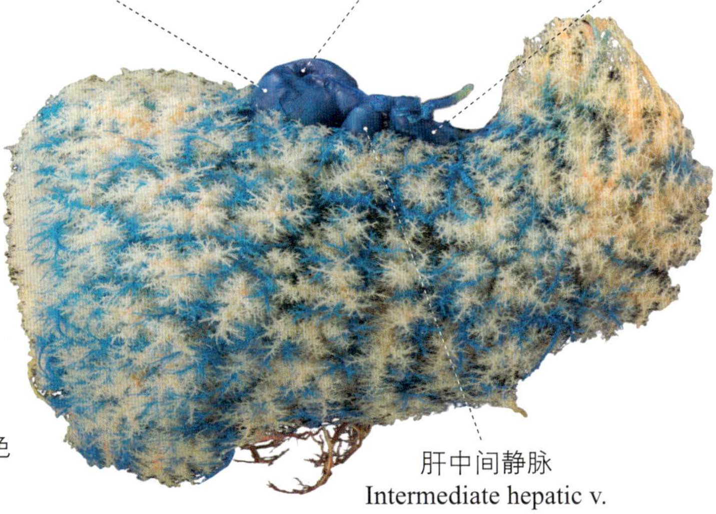

静脉—蓝色
肝门静脉分支—黄色
动脉—红色
Vein-blue colour
Branches of hepatic portal v.-yellow colour
Artery-red colour

图 2–28　肝的血管铸型
Cast of hepatic blood vessels

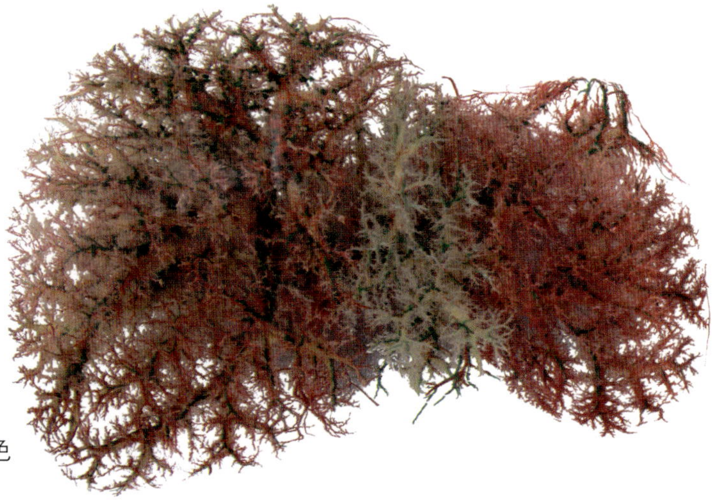

胆管—绿色
肝门静脉分支—黄色
动脉—红色
Bile duct-green colour
Branches of hepatic portal v.-yellow colour
Artery-red colour

图 2–29　肝的管道铸型（前面观）
Cast of hepatic vessels and ducts. Anterior aspect

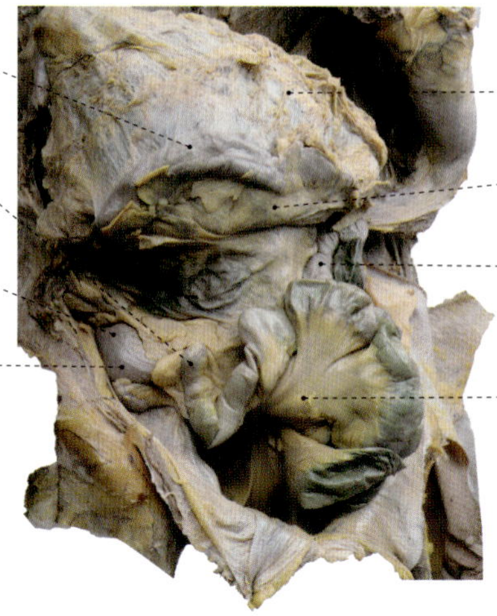

图 2-34　肠系膜与横结肠系膜

Mesentery and transverse mesocolon

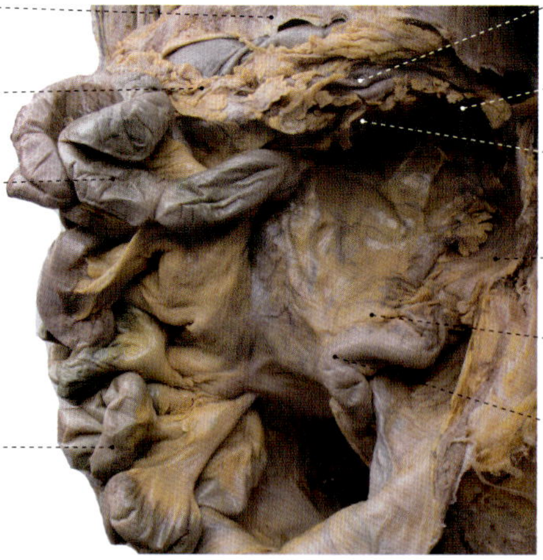

图 2-35　乙状结肠系膜

Sigmoid mesocolon

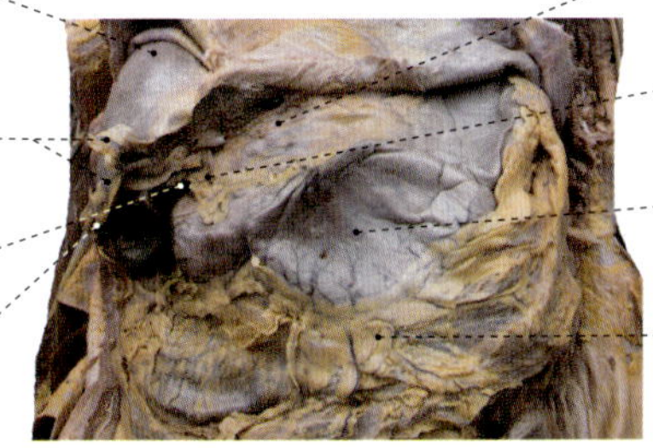

图 2-36 小网膜

Lesser omentum

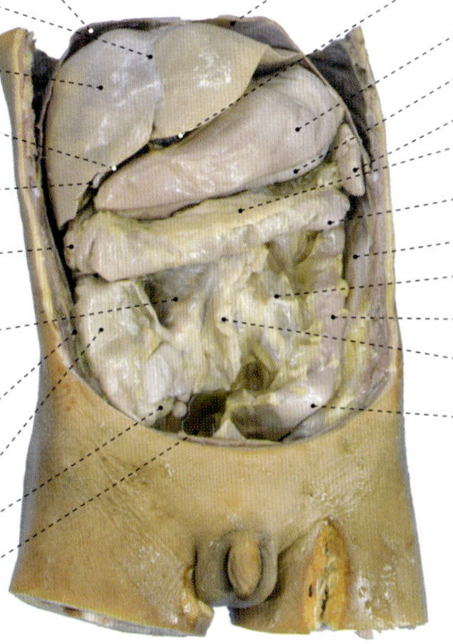

图 2-37 腹膜腔的交通

Communication of peritoneal cavity

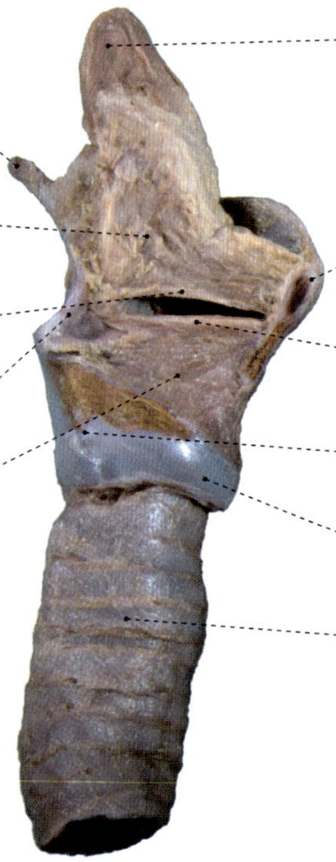

图 3-22　弹性圆锥和方形膜（外侧面观）

Conus elasticus and quadrangular membrane. Lateral aspect

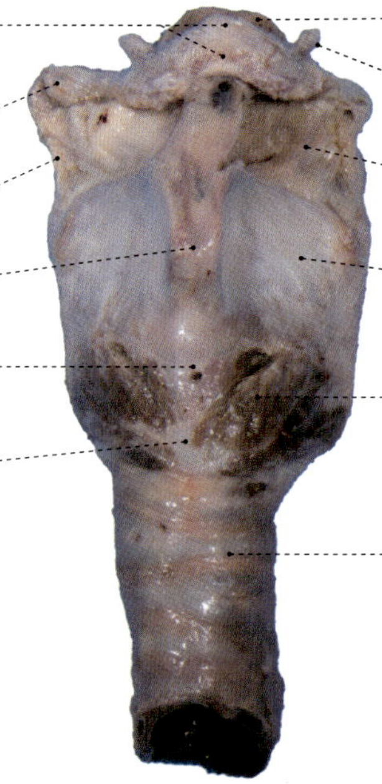

图 3-23　喉肌（前面观）

Muscles of larynx. Anterior aspect

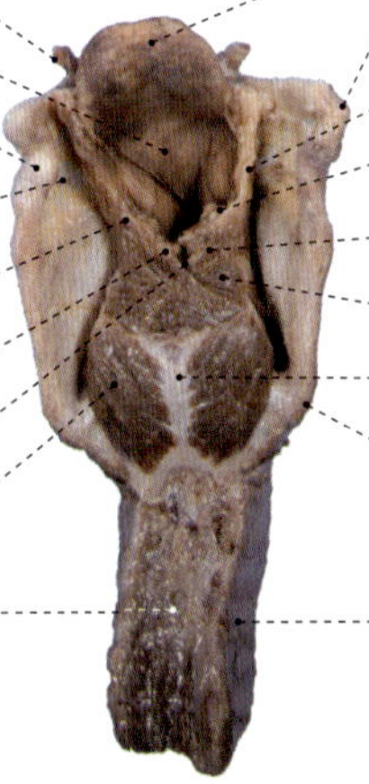

图 3–24　喉肌（后面观）

Muscles of larynx. Posterior aspect

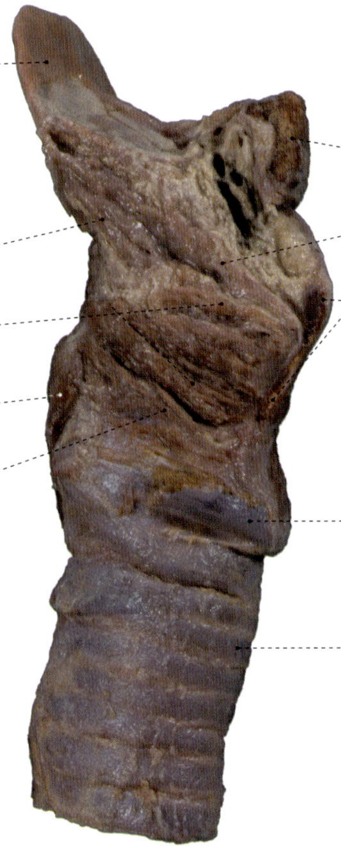

图 3–25　喉肌（外侧面观）

Muscles of larynx. Lateral aspect

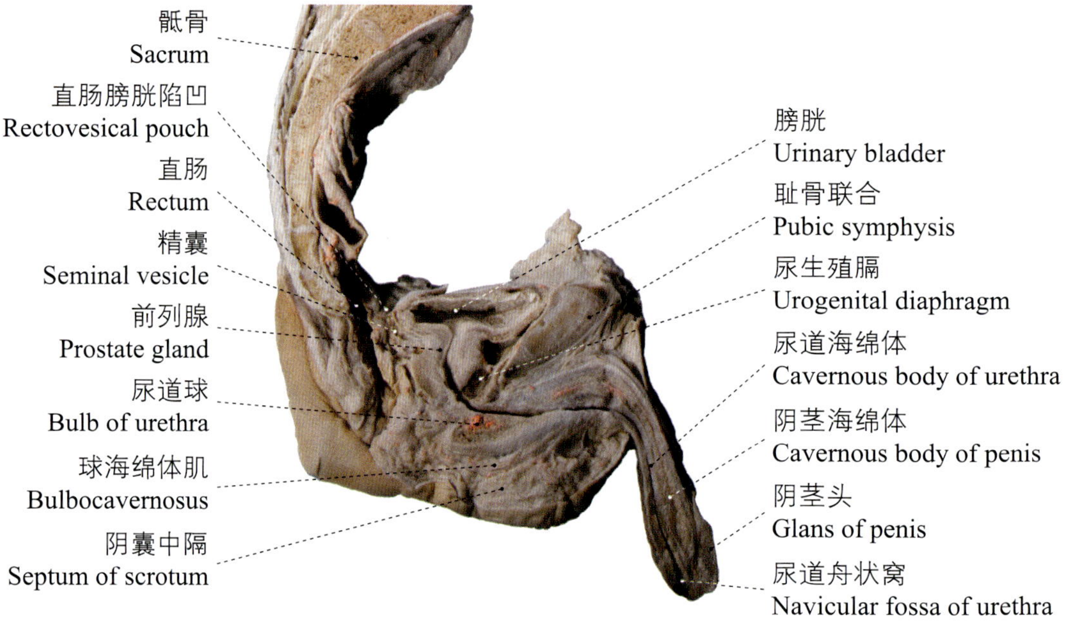

图 4–13 男性盆部（正中矢状切面）

Pelvis of male. Median saggital section

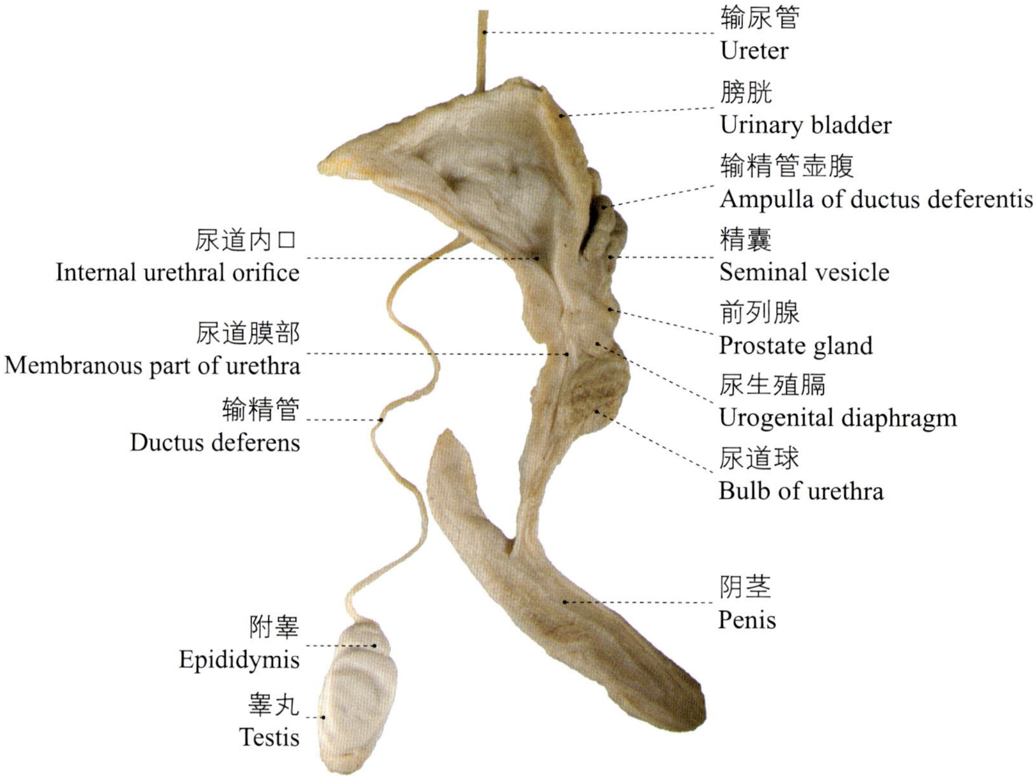

图 4–14 膀胱和男性生殖器（外侧面观）

Urinary bladder and male genital organs. Lateral aspect

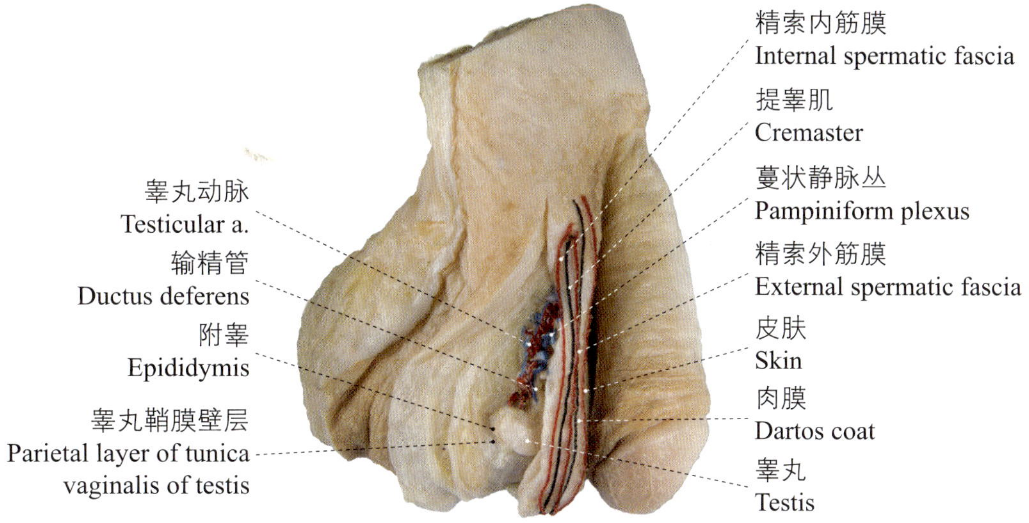

图 4–15　睾丸和精索被膜

Coverings of testis and spermatic cord

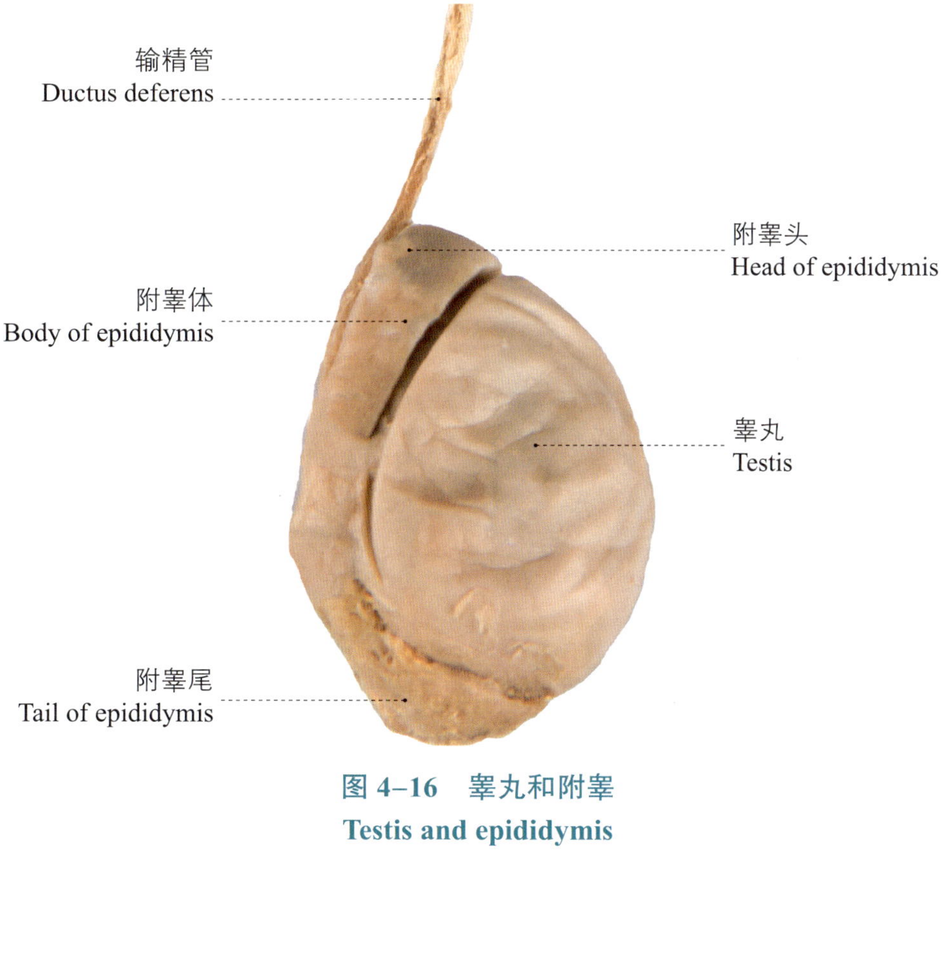

图 4–16　睾丸和附睾

Testis and epididymis

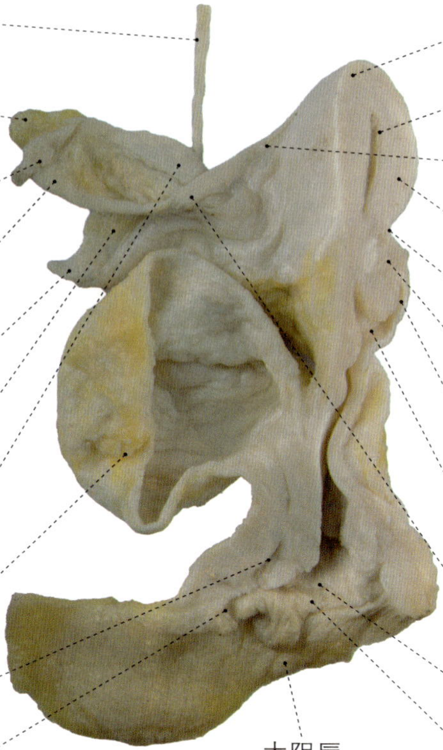

图 4–21　女性生殖系统（矢状切面）
Female genital system. Sagittal section

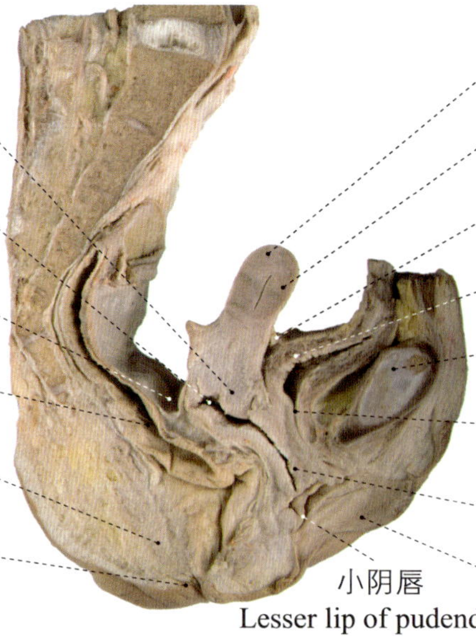

图 4–22　女性盆部（正中矢状切面）
Pelvis of female. Median sagittal section

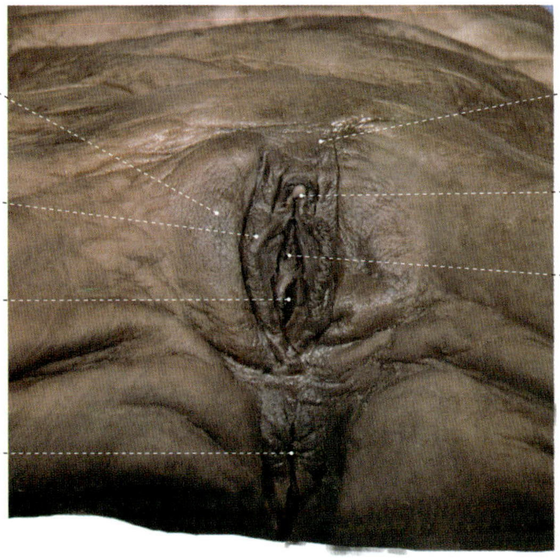

图 4–23　女性外生殖器

Female external genital organs

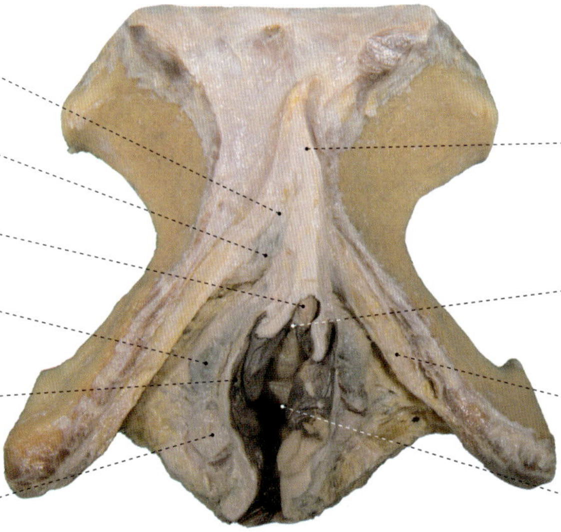

图 4–24　阴蒂、前庭球和前庭大腺（1）

Clitoris, bulb of vestibule and greater vestibular gland (1)

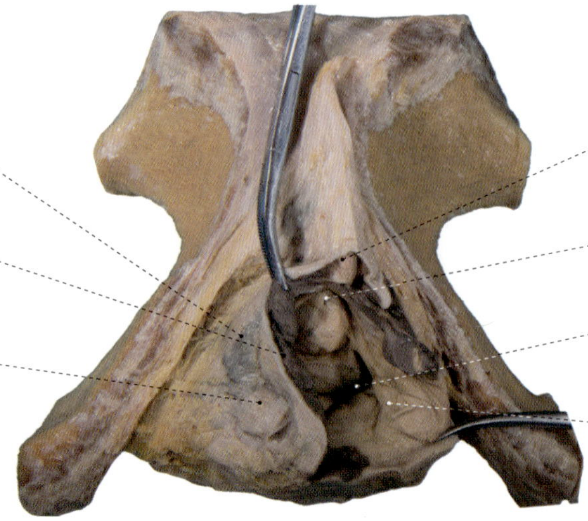

图 4–25　阴蒂、前庭球和前庭大腺（2）
Clitoris, bulb of vestibule and greater vestibular gland (2)

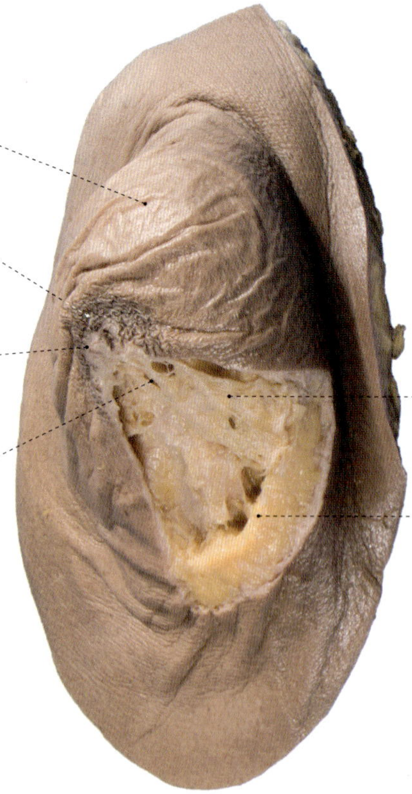

图 4–26　乳房（1）
Mamma (1)

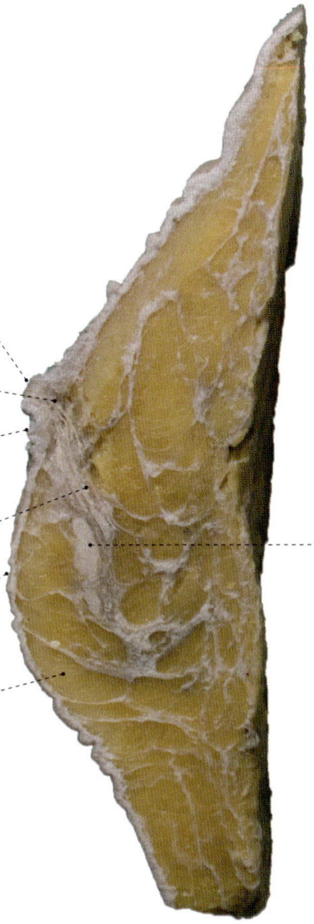

图 4–27　乳房（矢状切面）（2）
Mamma. Sagittal section (2)

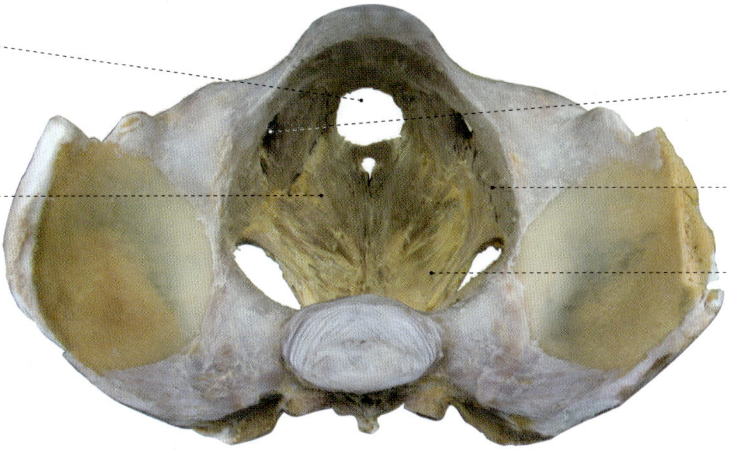

图 4–28　盆底肌
Muscles of pelvic floor

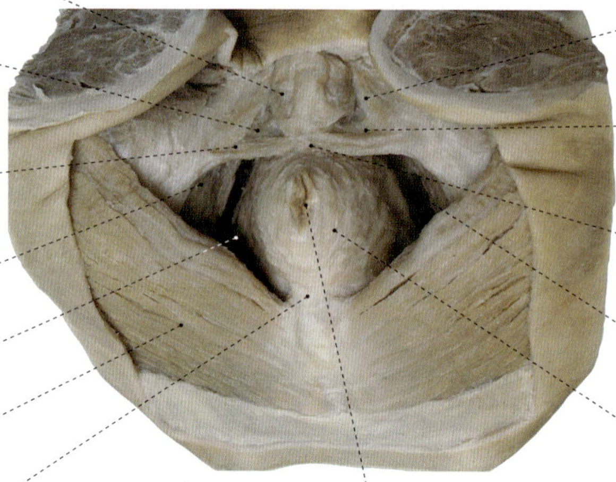

图 4–29　男性会阴肌

Muscles of male perineum

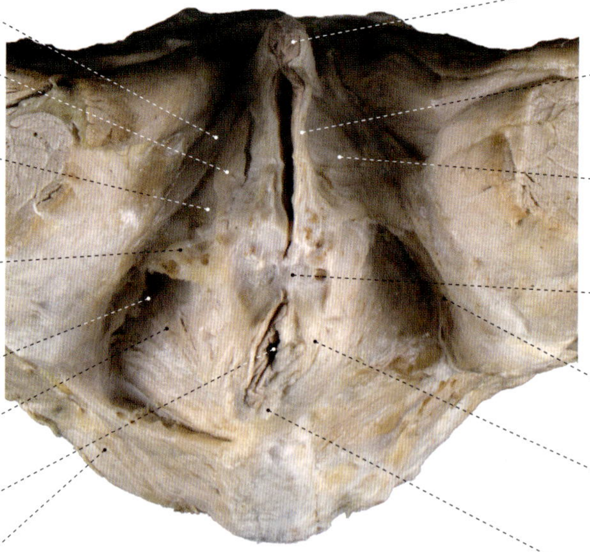

图 4–30　女性会阴肌

Muscles of female perineum

第五章　心

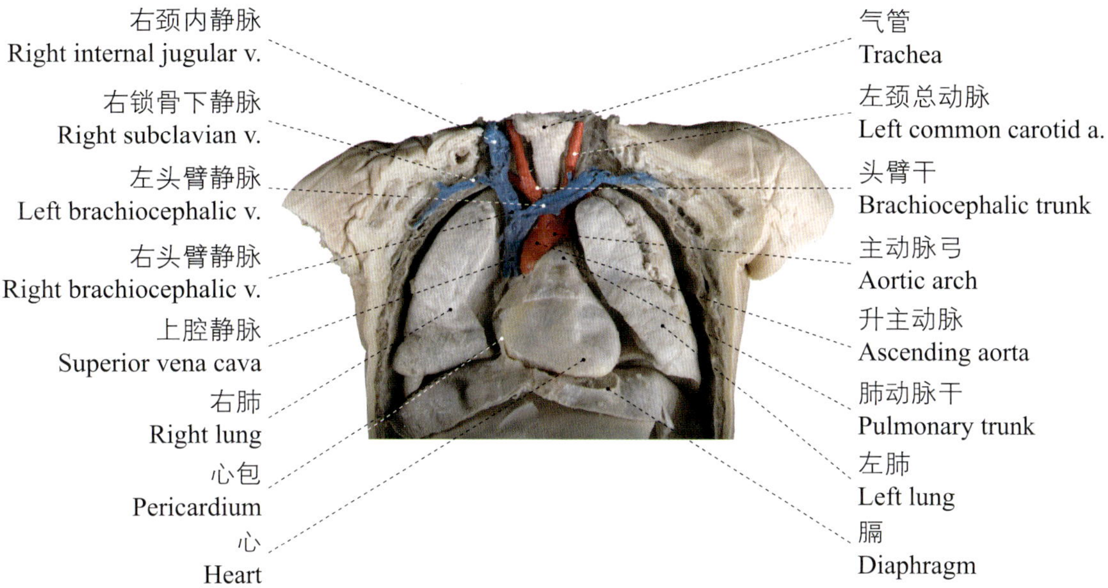

图 5-1　心的位置

Position of heart

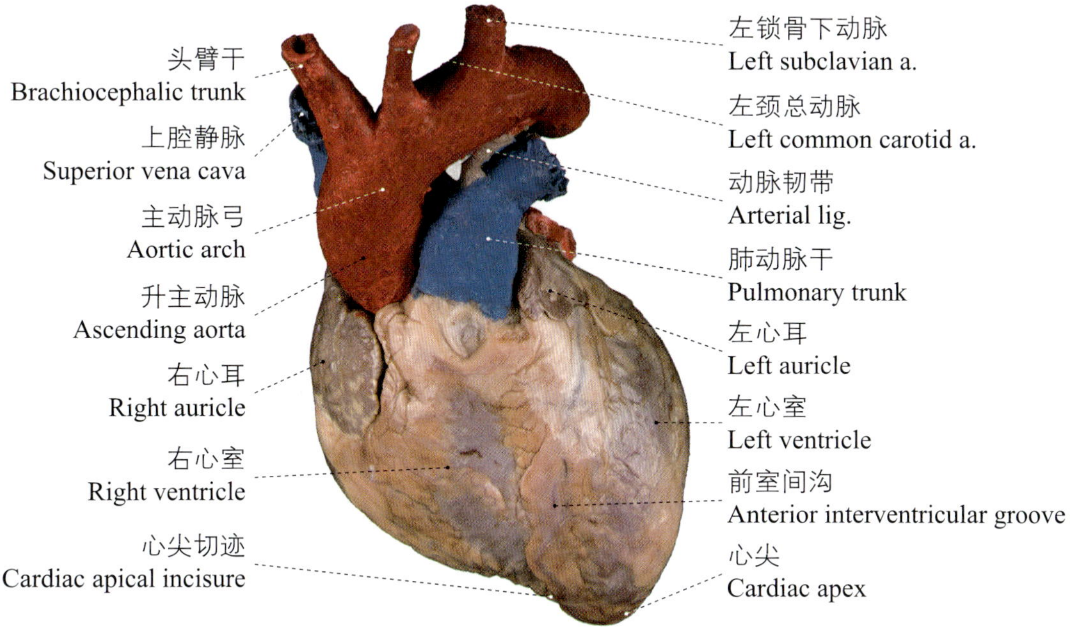

图 5-2　心脏的外形（前面观）

External features of heart. Anterior aspect

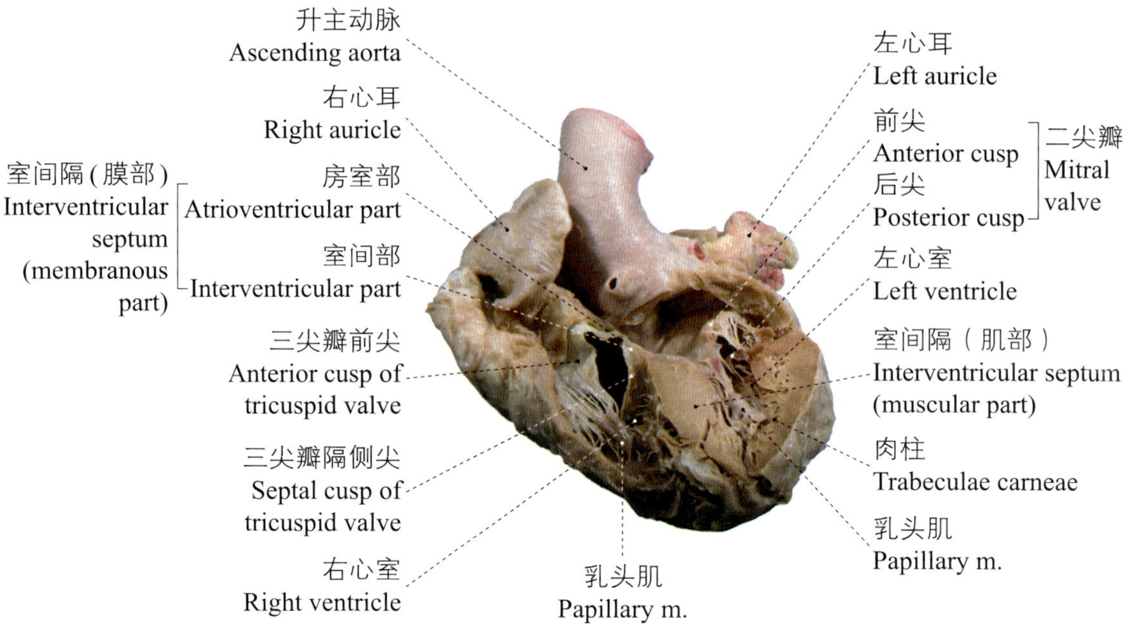

图 5–7　心的内腔

Internal cavities of the heart

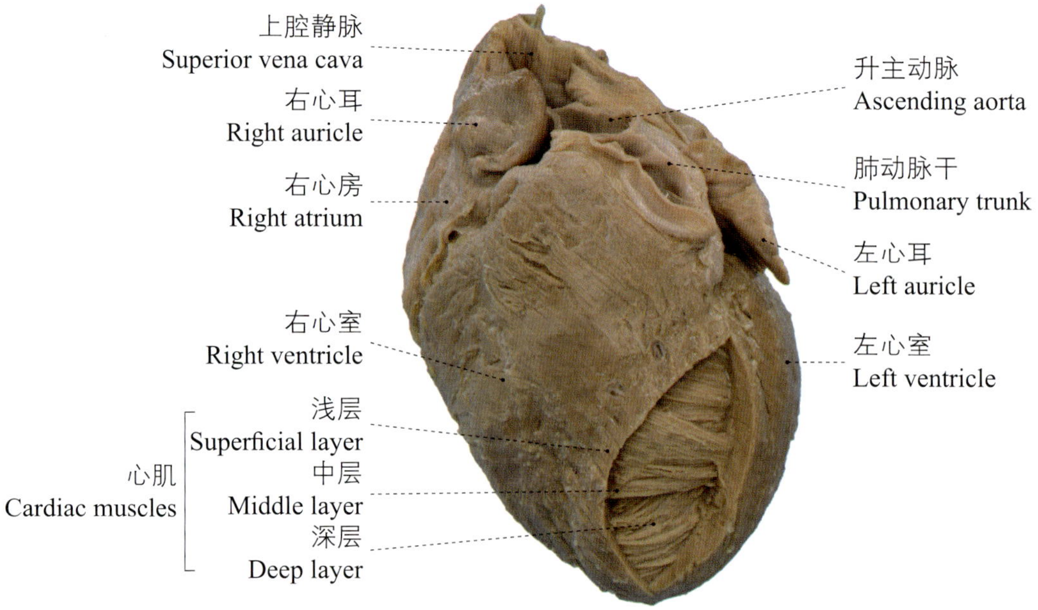

图 5–8　心肌的走行

Course of cardiac muscles

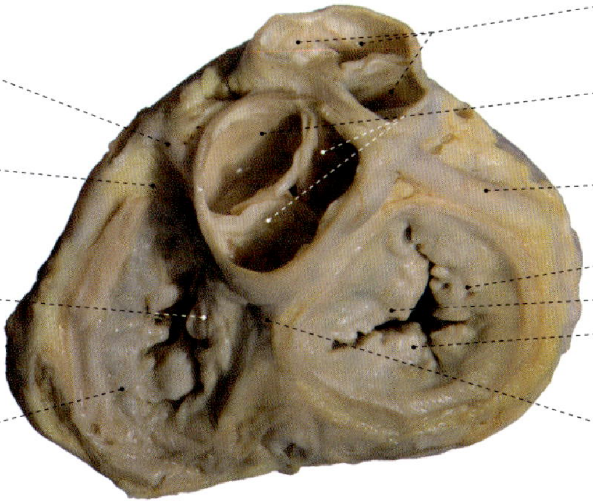

图 5-9　心瓣膜

Valves of heart

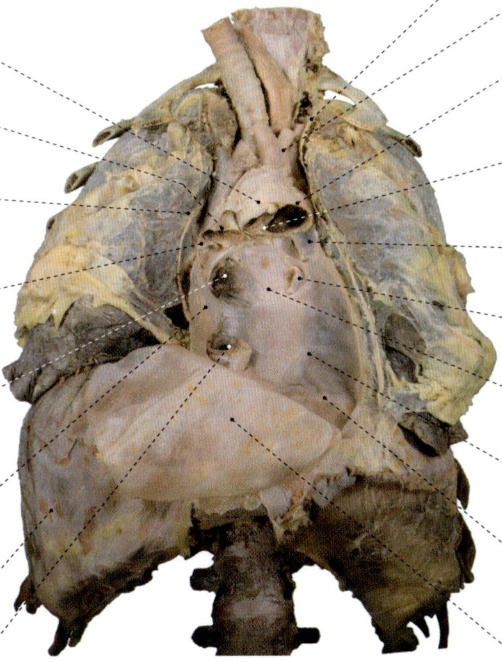

图 5-10　心包（心脏已切除）

Pericardium. Heart removed

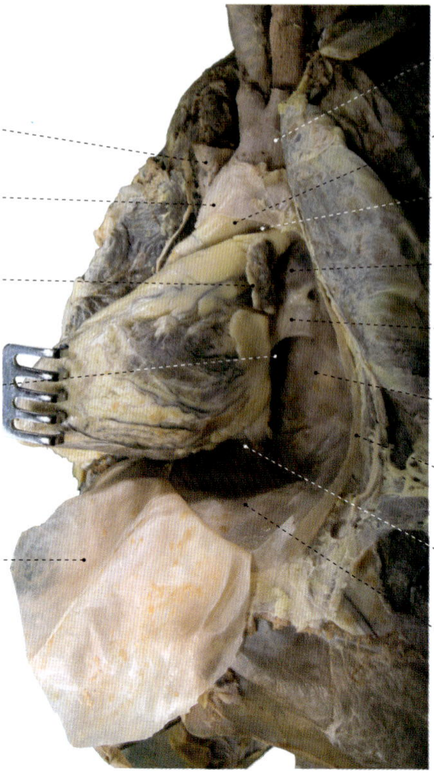

图 5-11　心被从打开的心包中拉出（左侧面观）

Heart drawn out of opened pericardium. Left lateral view

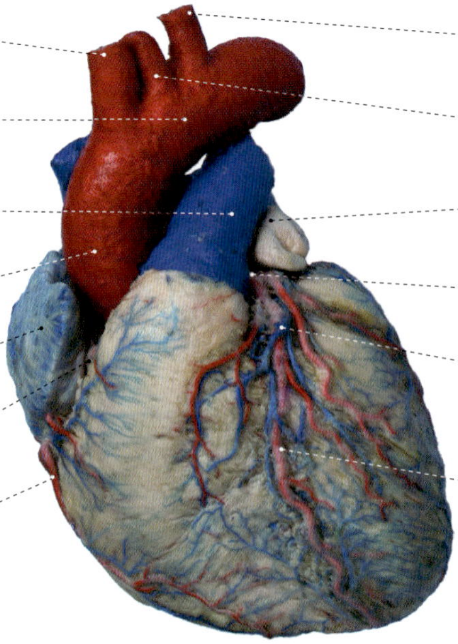

图 5-12　心的血管（前面观）

Blood vessels of heart. Anterior aspect

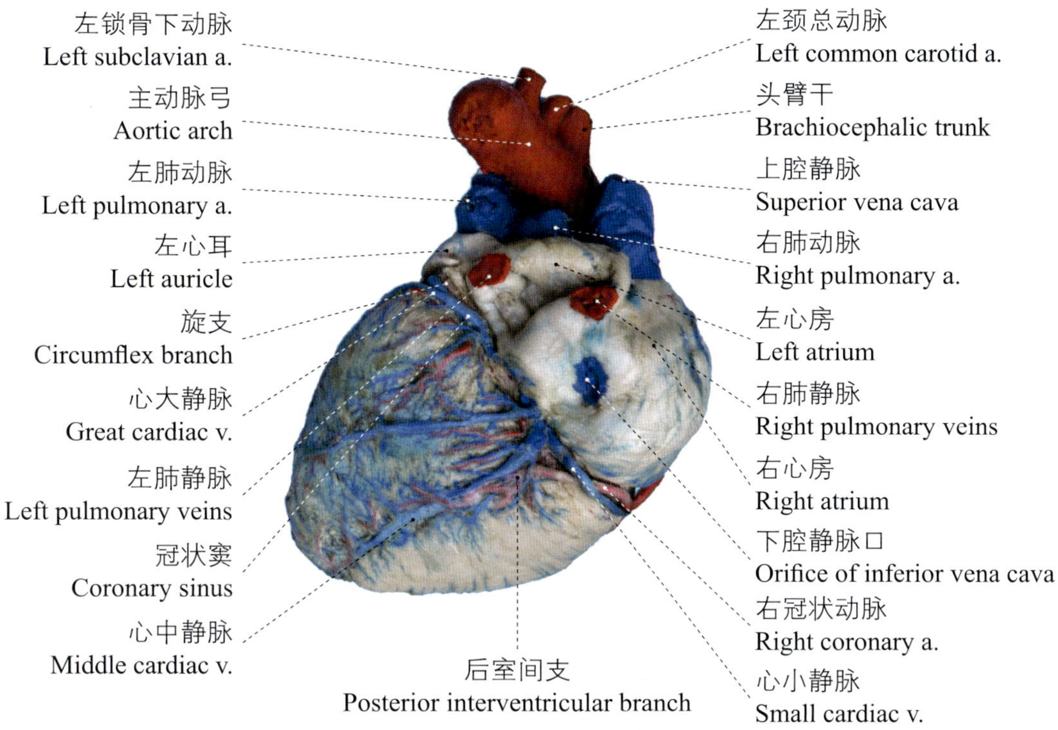

图 5-13 心的血管（后面观）

Blood vessels of heart. Posterior aspect

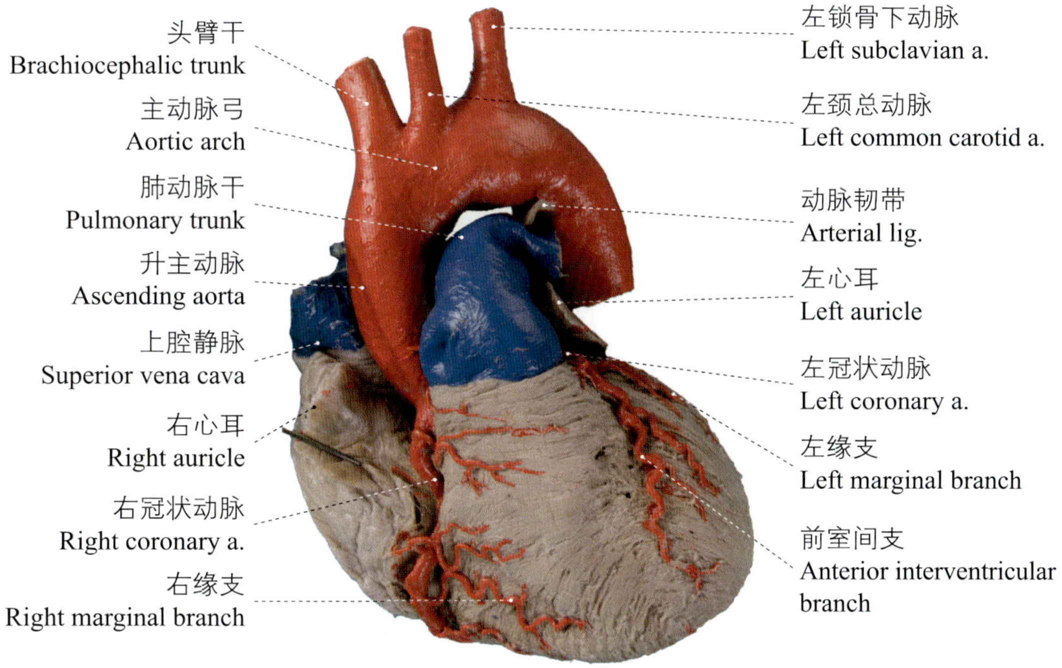

图 5-14 心的动脉（前面观）

Arteries of heart. Anterior aspect

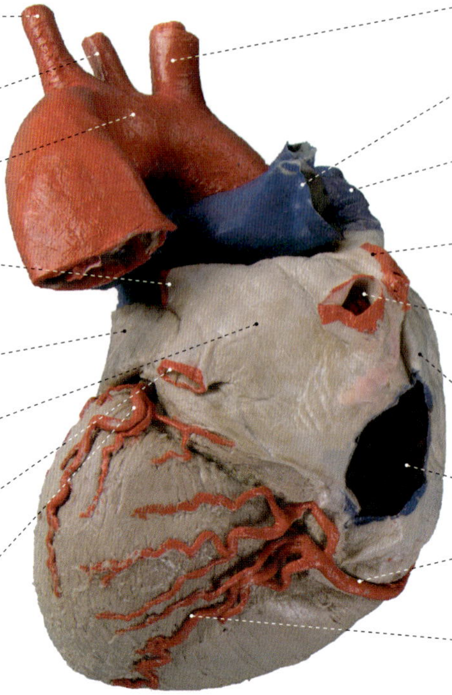

图 5-15　心的动脉（后面观）

Arteries of heart. Posterior aspect

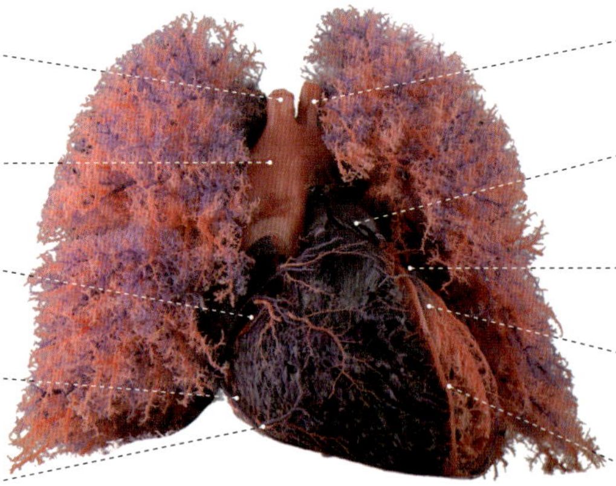

心：右半心和静脉—紫色 左半心和动脉—红色
Heart: right half and vein—purple colour left half and vein—red colour
肺：肺动脉—紫色 肺静脉—红色
Lung: pulmonary artery—purple colour pulmonary vein—red colour

图 5-16　心和肺的血管铸型标本

Cast of the blood vessels of heart and lungs

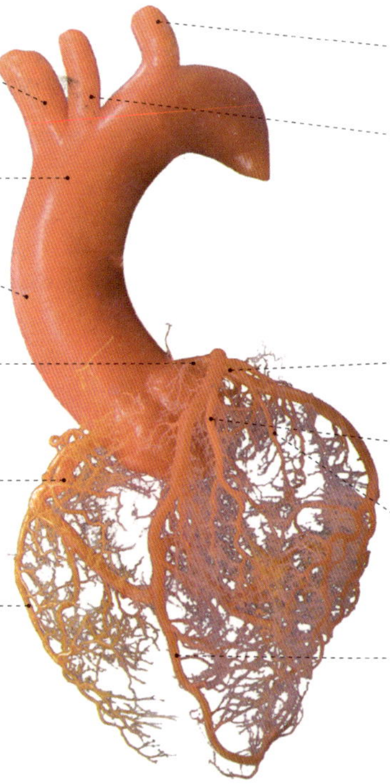

图 5–17 心动脉的铸型（前面观）（1）

Cast of cardiac arteries. Anterior aspect (1)

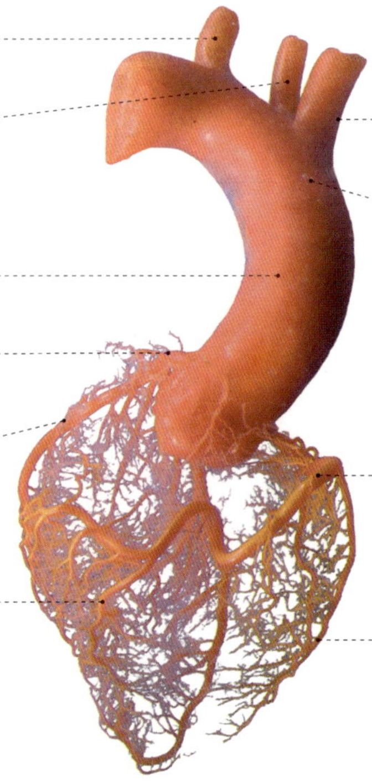

图 5–18 心动脉的铸型（后面观）（2）

Cast of cardiac arteries. Posterior aspect (2)

第六章 淋巴系统

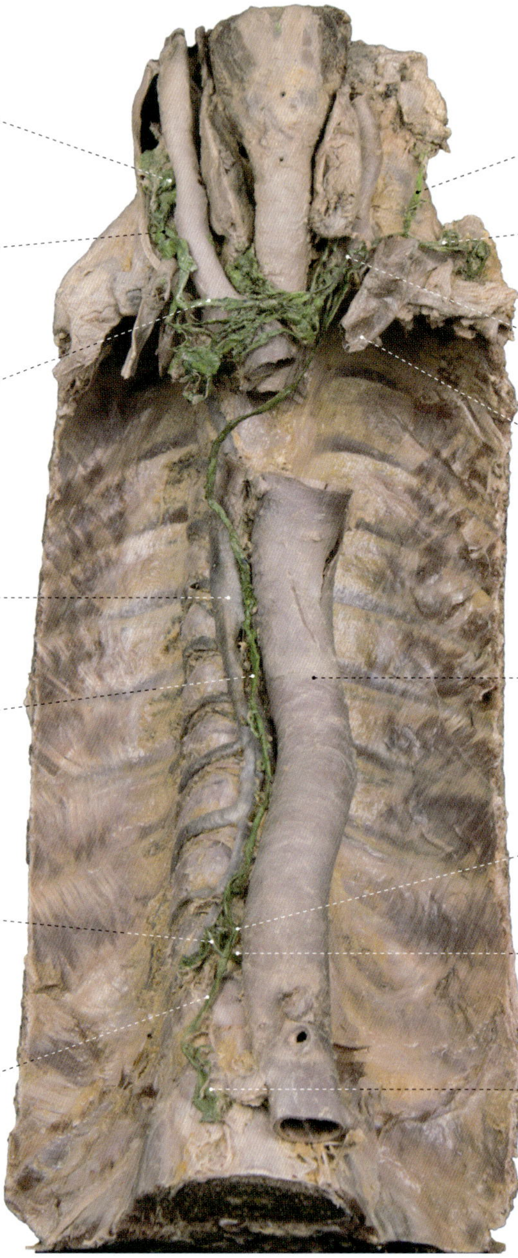

图 6-1 胸导管及淋巴干

Thoracic duct and lymphatic trunks

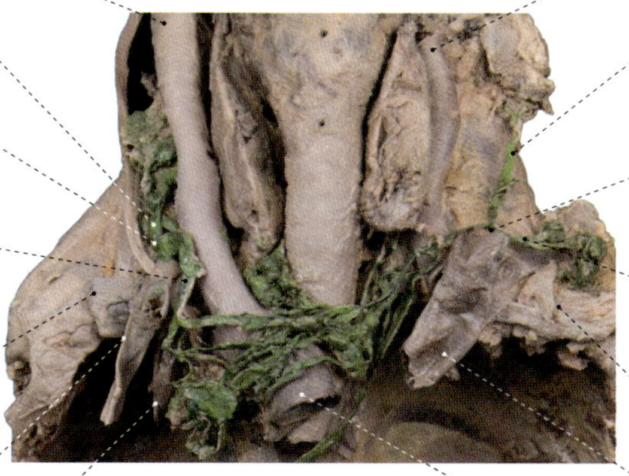

图 6–2　淋巴导管及淋巴干

Lymphatic ducts and trunks

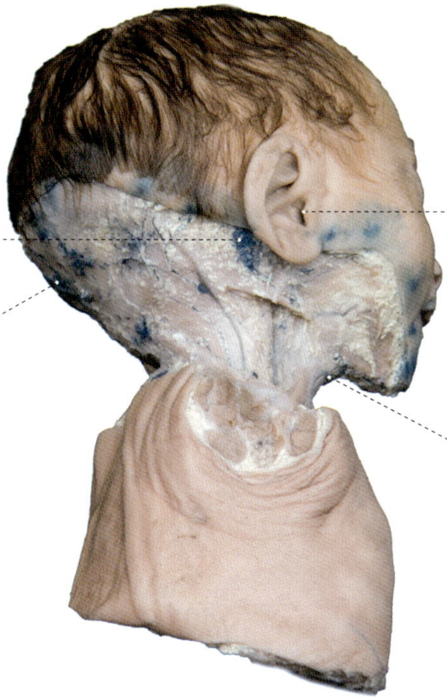

图 6–3　头颈部的淋巴管及淋巴结（1）

Lymphatic vessels and lymph nodes of head and neck (1)

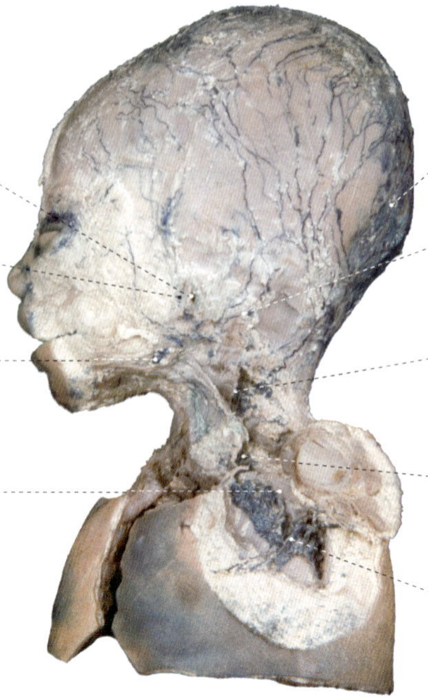

图 6-4　头颈部的淋巴管及淋巴结（2）

Lymphatic vessels and lymph nodes of the head and neck (2)

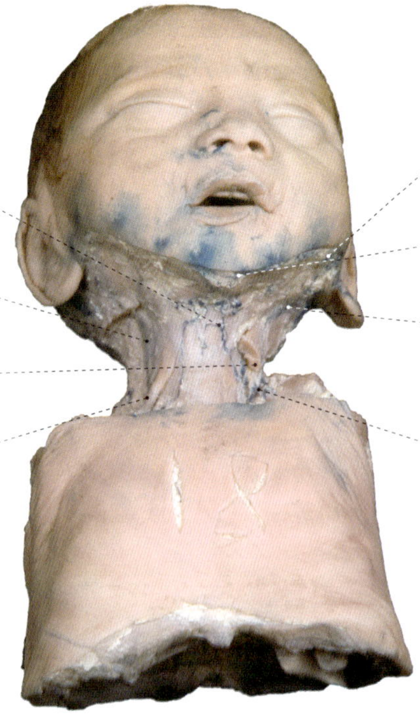

图 6-5　颈前部的淋巴管及淋巴结

Lymphatic vessels and lymph nodes of neck

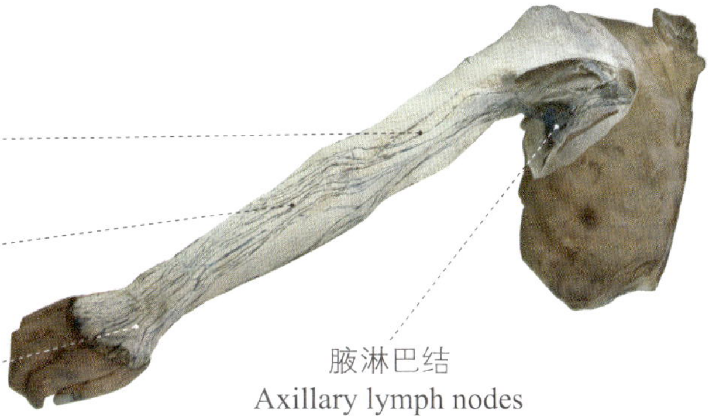

图 6–6 上肢的淋巴管及淋巴结

Lymphatic vessels and lymph nodes of upper limb

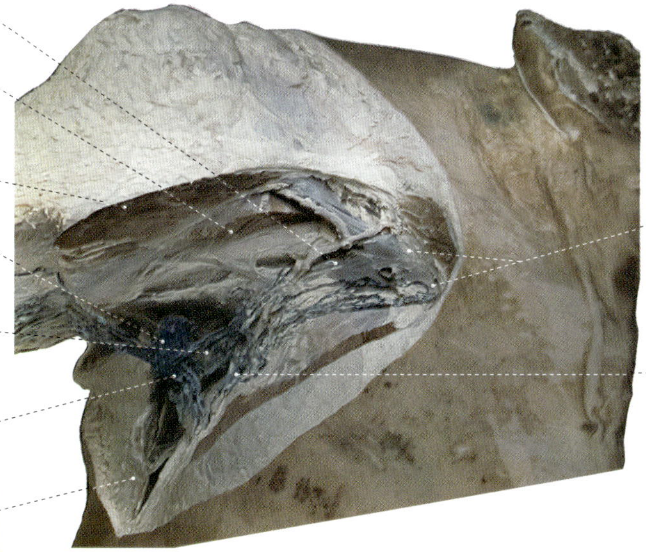

图 6–7 腋窝的淋巴管和淋巴结

Lymphatic vessels and lymph nodes of axillary fossa

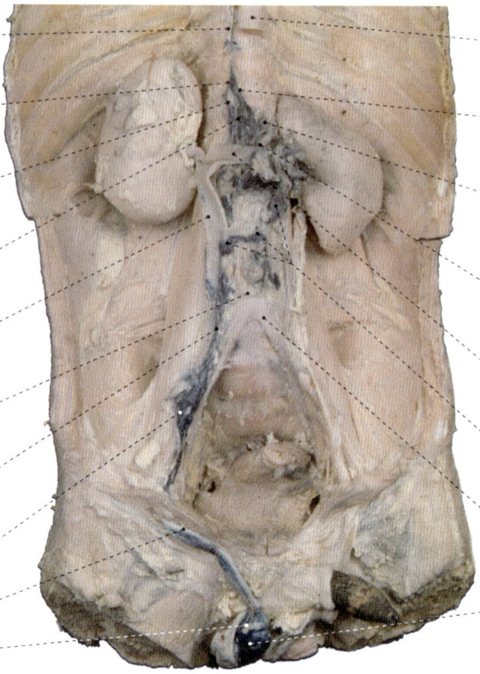

图 6–12　腹部器官的淋巴结（2）

Lymphatic vessels of stomach (2)

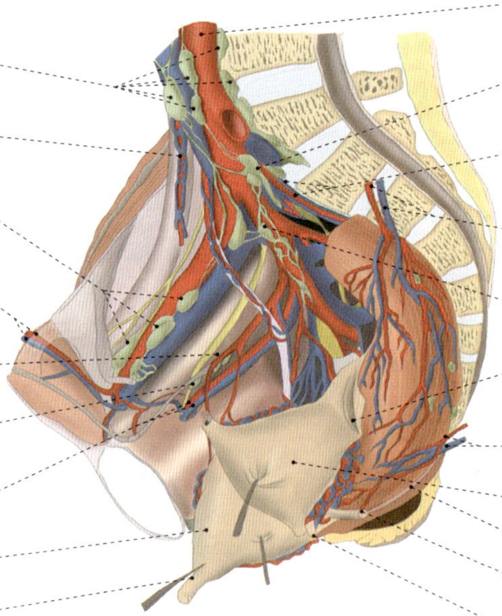

图 6–13　盆部的淋巴管和淋巴结（女性）

Lymphatic vessels and lymph nodes of pelvis (female)

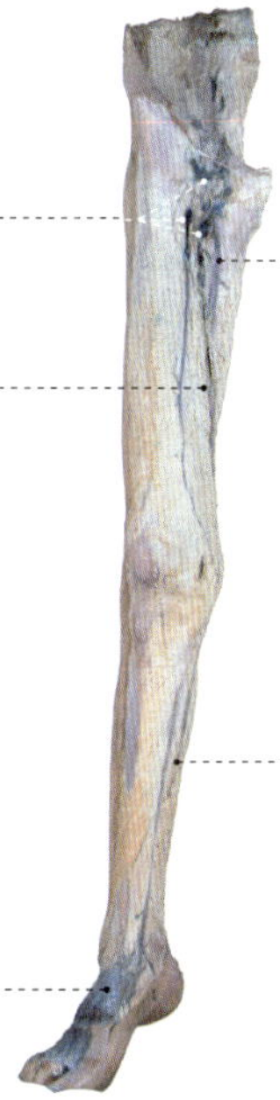

图 6–14　下肢的浅淋巴管和淋巴结

Superficial lymphatic vessels and lymph nodes of lower limb

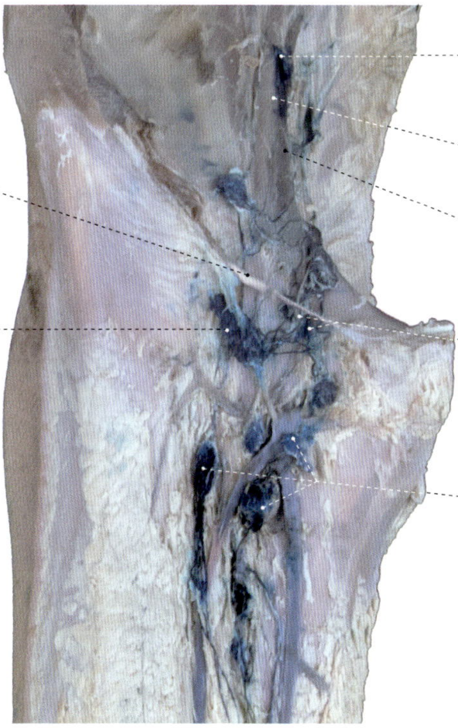

图 6–15　腹股沟淋巴结

Superficial inguinal lymph nodes

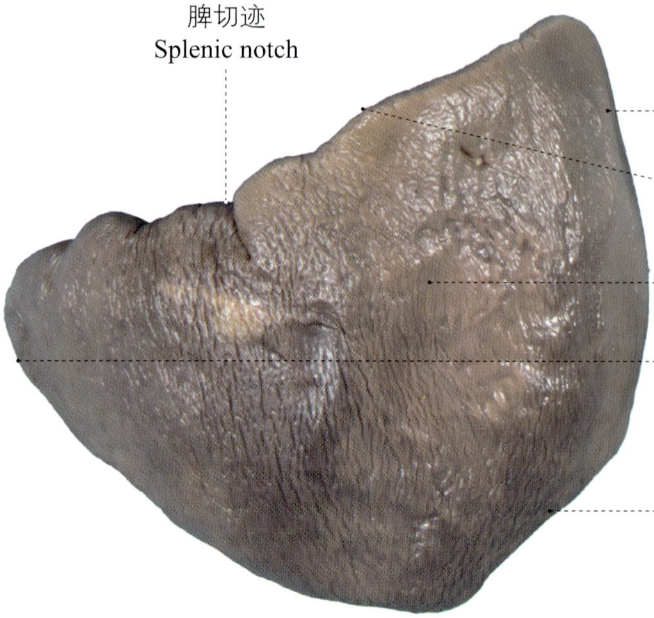

图 6–16　脾（膈面观）

Spleen. diaphragmatic aspect

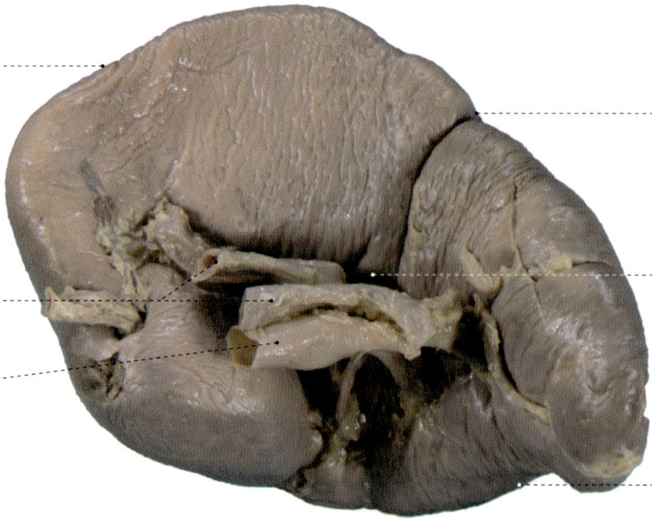

图 6–17　脾（脏面观）

Spleen. visceral aspect

第七章　感觉器

第一节　视　器

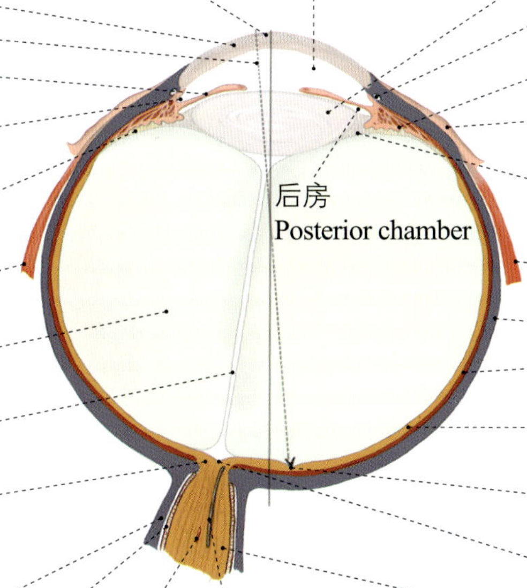

图 7–1　右侧眼球模式图（水平断面）

Diagram of right eyeball. Horizontal section

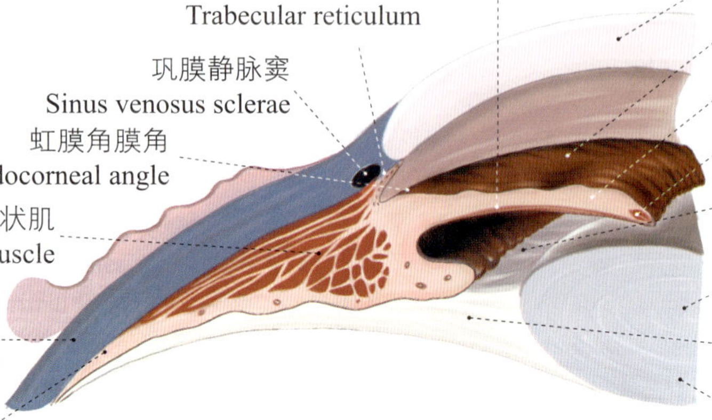

图 7–2　眼球前部的断面模式图

Diagram of section through anterior part of eyeball

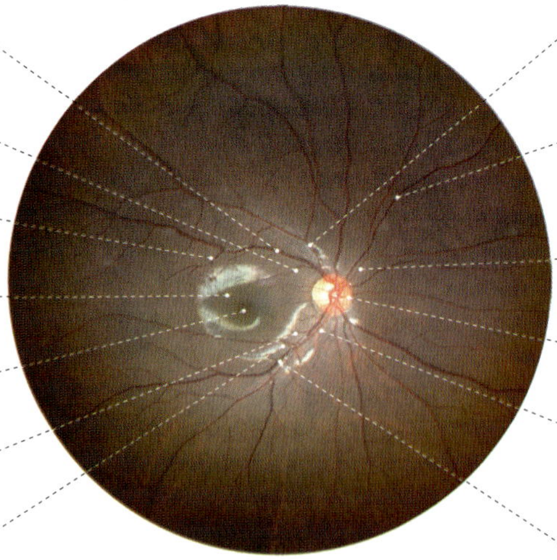

图 7–3　检眼镜所见（右侧）

Ophthalmoscopic view of fundus of eyeball. Right side

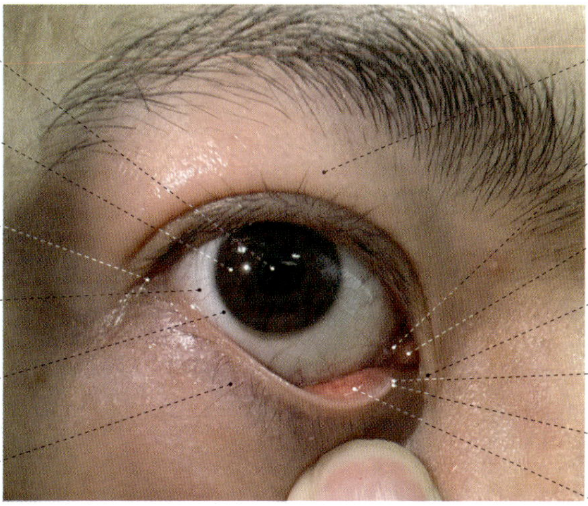

图 7-4 右眼（前面观）
Right eye. Anterior aspect

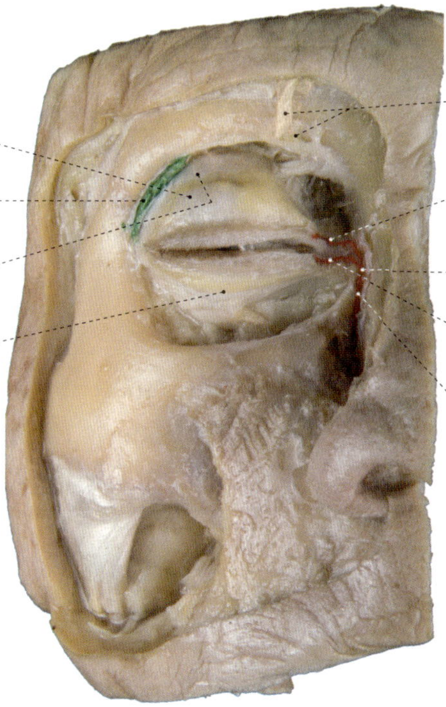

图 7-5 泪器（1）
Lacrimal apparatus (1)

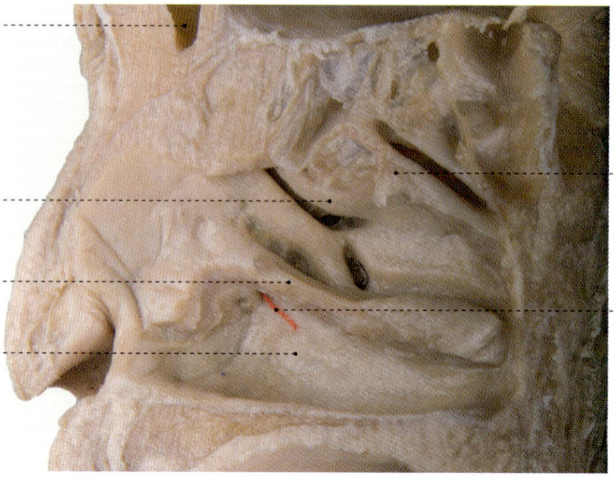

图 7–6　泪器（2）

Lacrimal apparatus (2)

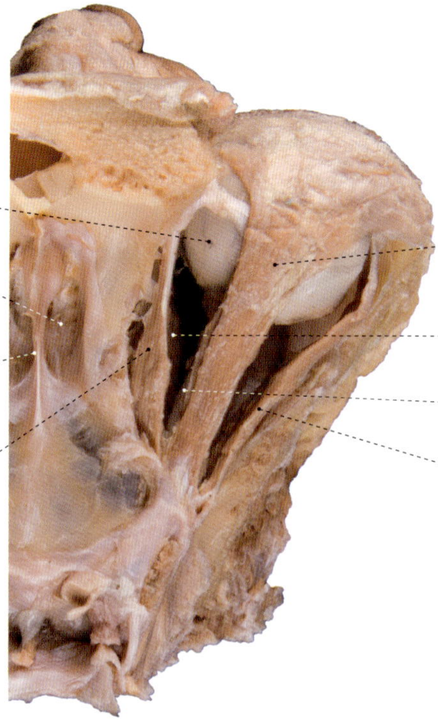

图 7–7　眼球外肌（上面观）

Extraocular muscles. Superior aspect

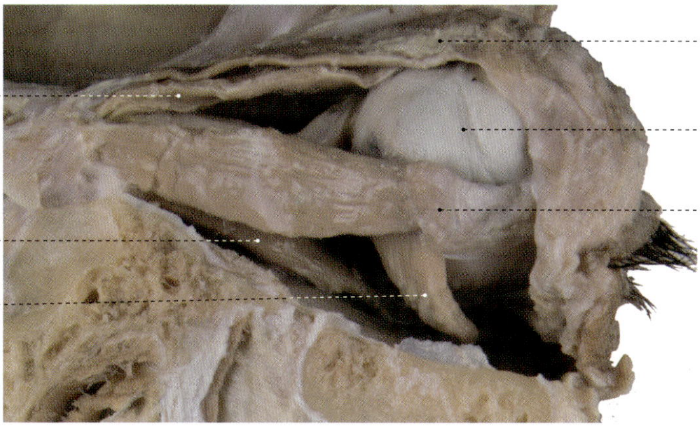

图 7–8 眼球外肌（外侧面观）
Exterocular muscles. Lateral aspect

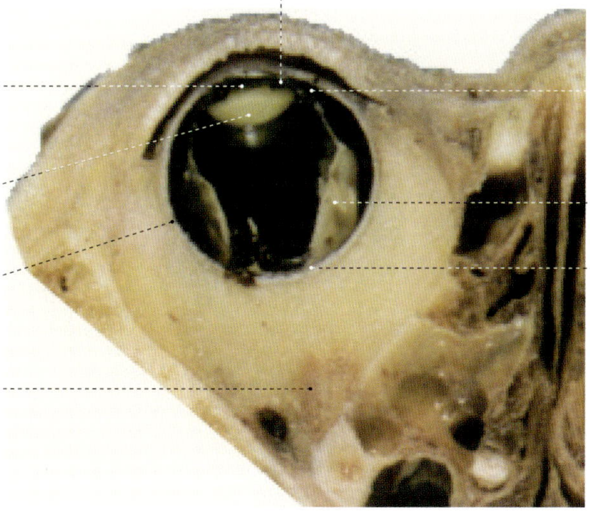

图 7–9 右眶（水平切面）（下面观）
Right orbit. Horizontal section. Inferior aspect

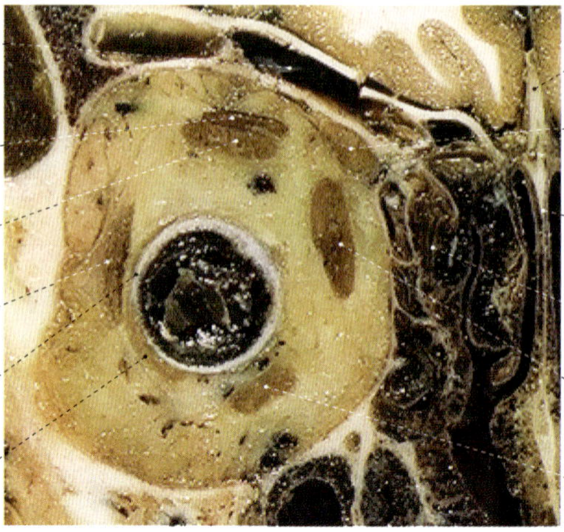

图 7-10　右眶（冠状切面）

Right orbit. Coronal section

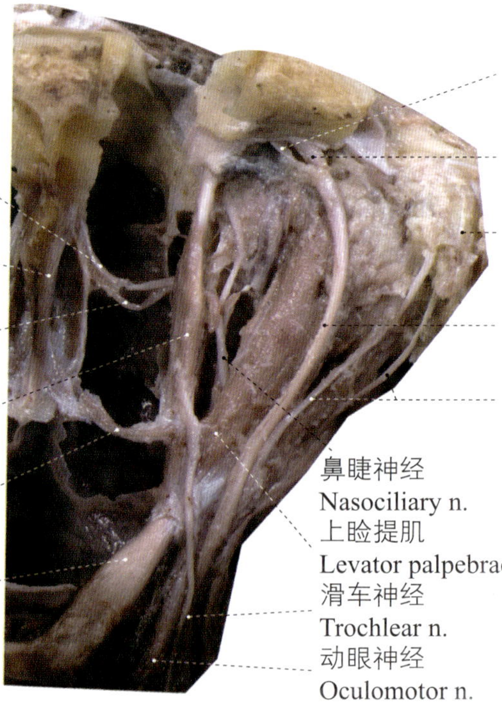

图 7-11　眼的血管、神经（上面观）

Blood vessels and nerves of eye. Superior aspect

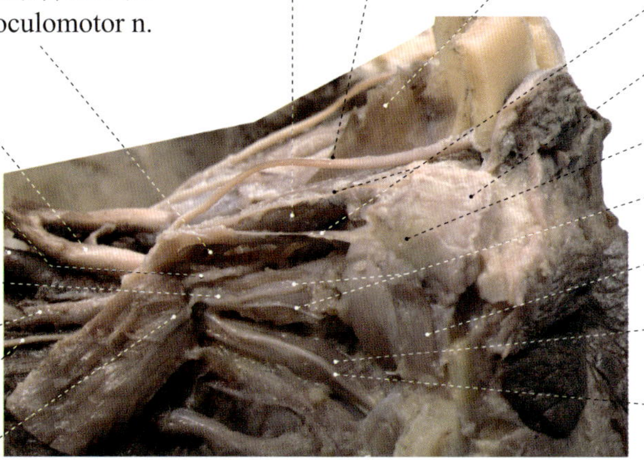

图 7–12　眼的肌肉、血管、神经（外侧面观）

Muscles, blood vessels and nerves of eye. Lateral aspect

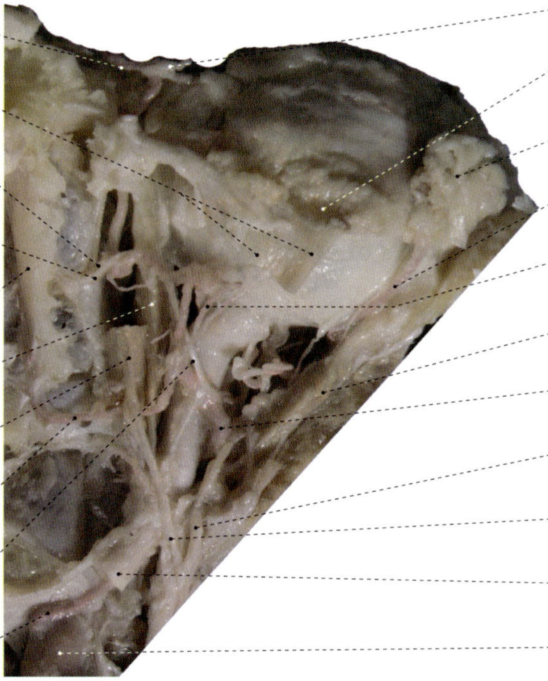

图 7–13　眼的动脉（上面观）

Arteres of the eye. Superior aspect

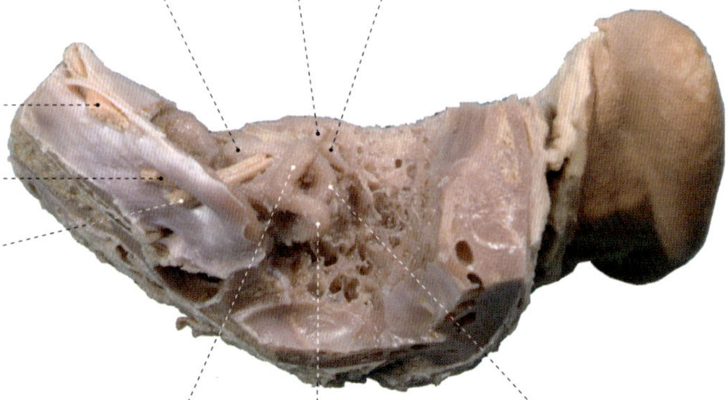

图 7-17　前庭蜗器概观（后上面观）

General arrangement of vestibulocochlear organ. Posterosuperior aspect

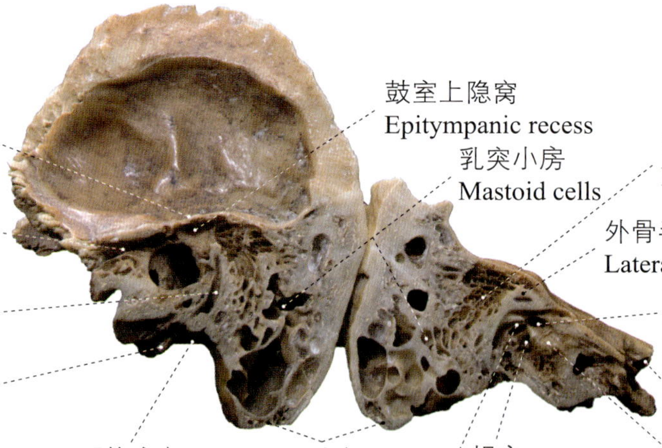

图 7-18　打开的颞骨

Temporal bone is opened

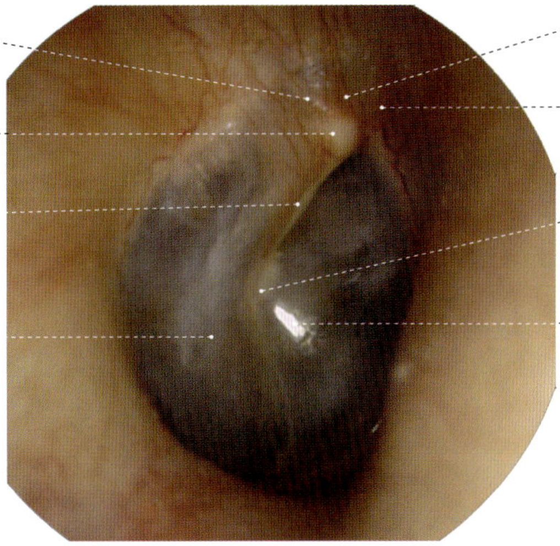

图 7–19　鼓膜耳镜所见
Otoscopic view of the tympanic membrane

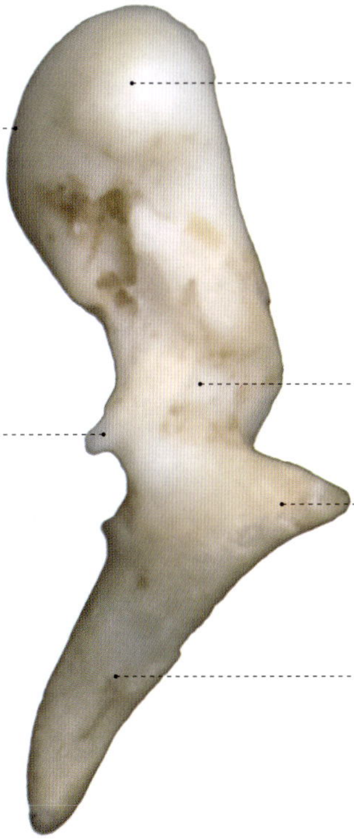

图 7–20　锤骨（外侧面观）
Malleus. Lateral aspect

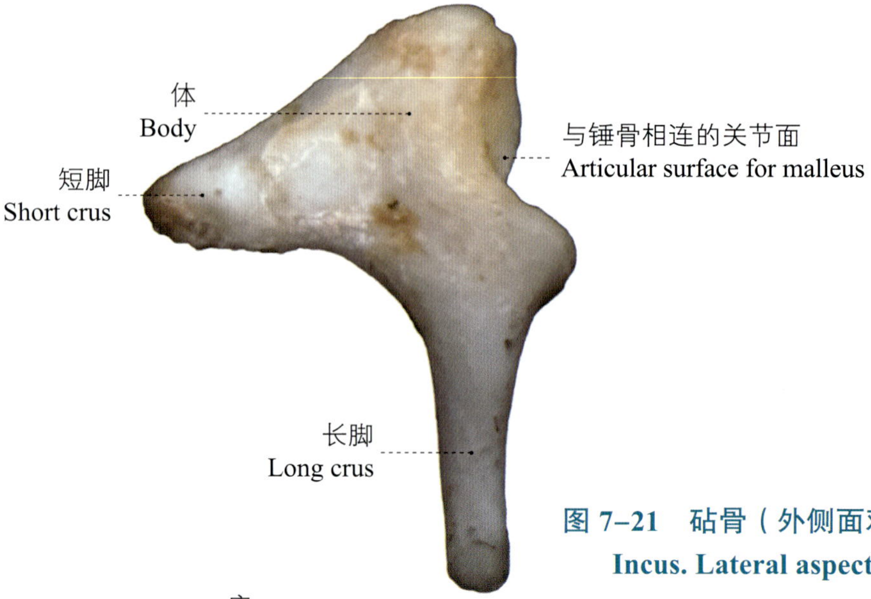

图 7–21　砧骨（外侧面观）
Incus. Lateral aspect

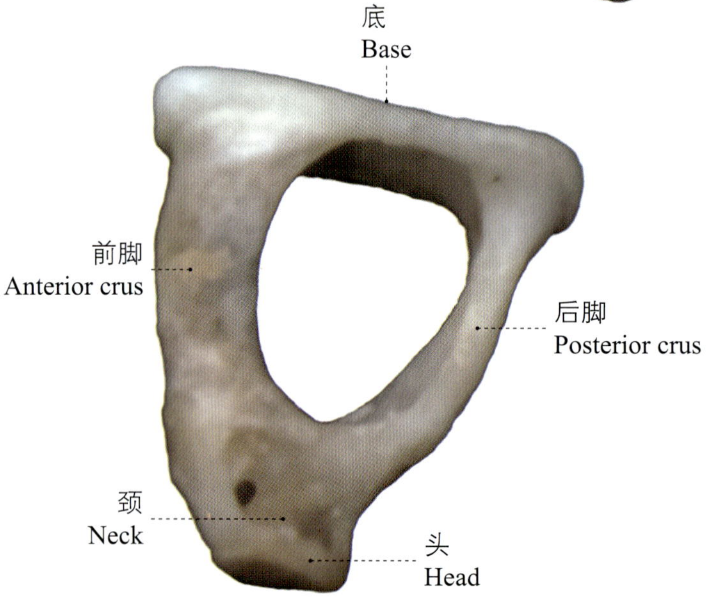

图 7–22　镫骨（上外侧面观）
Stapes. Superolateral aspect

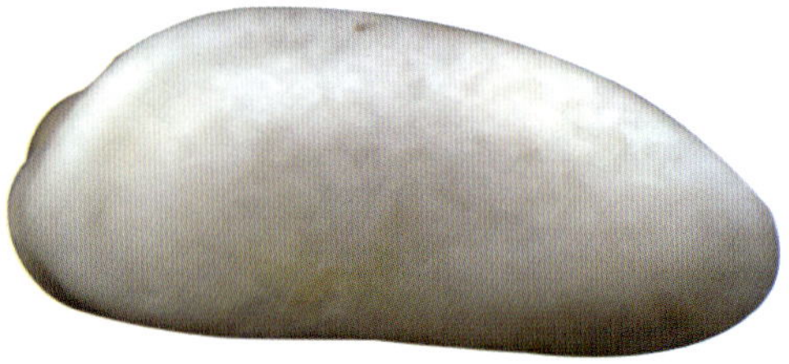

图 7–23　镫骨底
Base of stapes

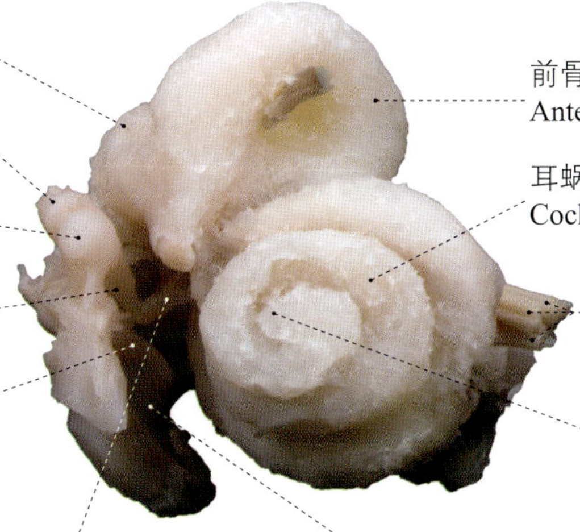

图 7–24　鼓膜、听小骨链和骨迷路（前外上面观）

Tympanic membrane, chain of the auditory ossicles and bony labyrinth. Anterosuperior and lateral aspect

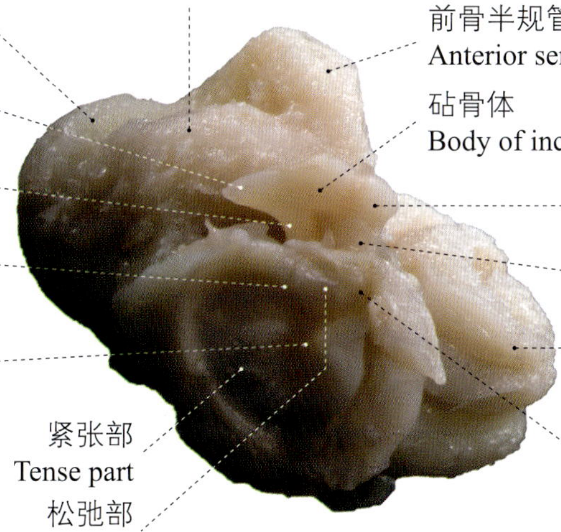

图 7–25　鼓膜、听小骨和骨迷路（外侧面观）

Tympanic membrane, auditory ossicles and bony labyrinth. Lateral aspect

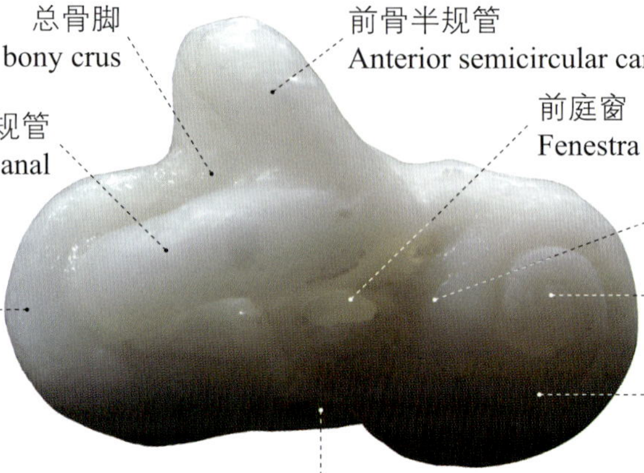

图 7–26　骨迷路（前外侧面观）

Bony labyrinth of right ear. Anterolateral aspect

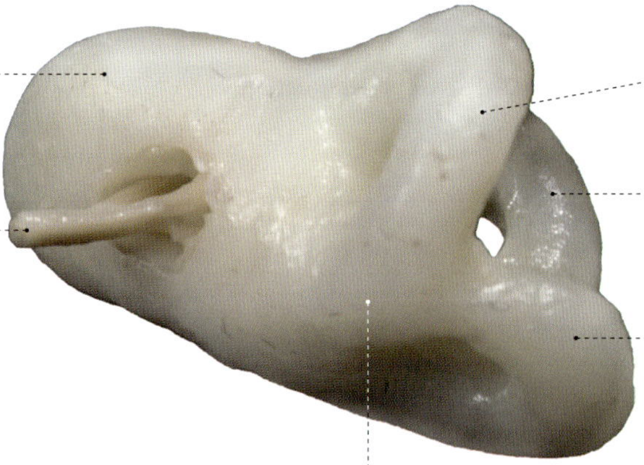

图 7–27　右耳骨迷路（后内侧面观）

Bony labyrinth of right ear. Posteromedial aspect

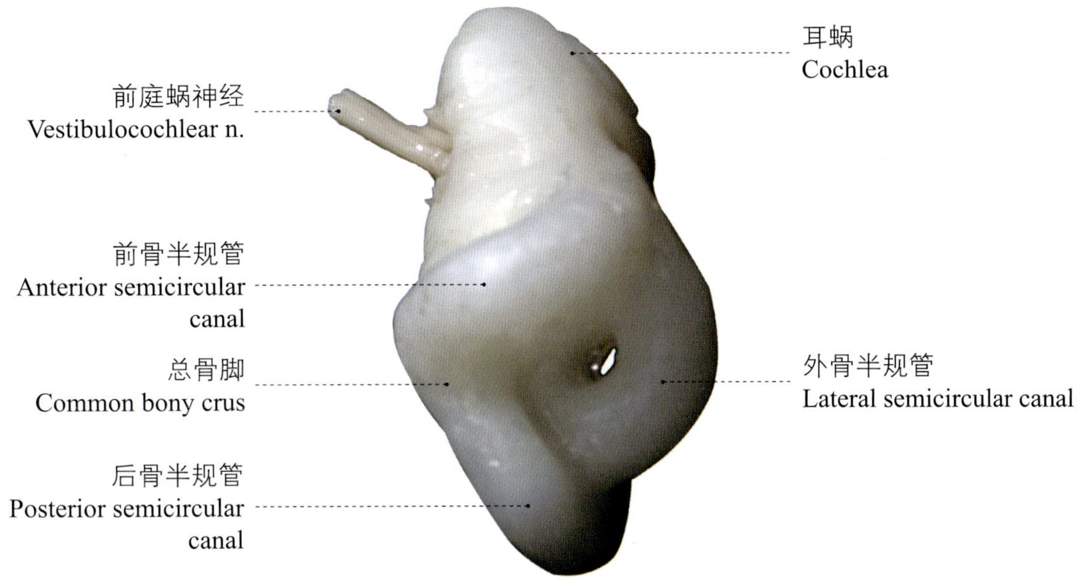

图 7–28 右耳骨迷路（上面观）
Bony labyrinth of right ear. Superior aspect

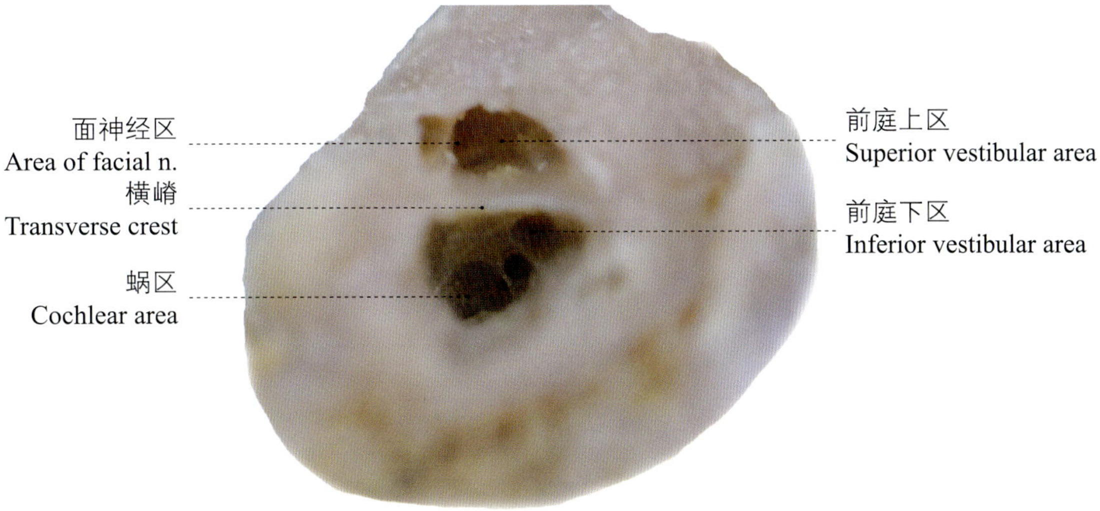

图 7–29 内耳道底
Fundus of internal acoustic meatus

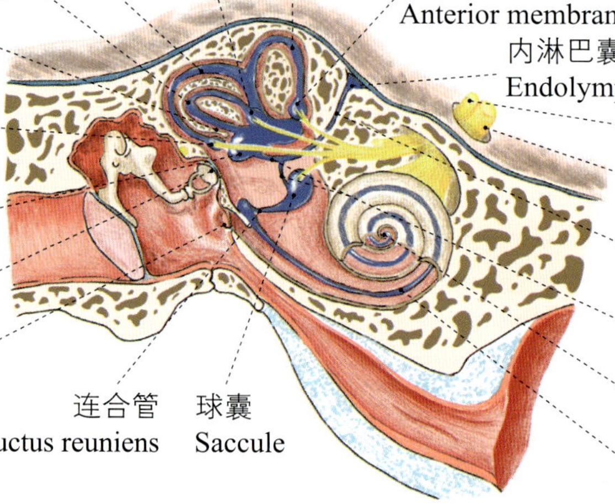

图 7-30 骨迷路与膜迷路模式图

Diagram of bony and membranous labyrinth

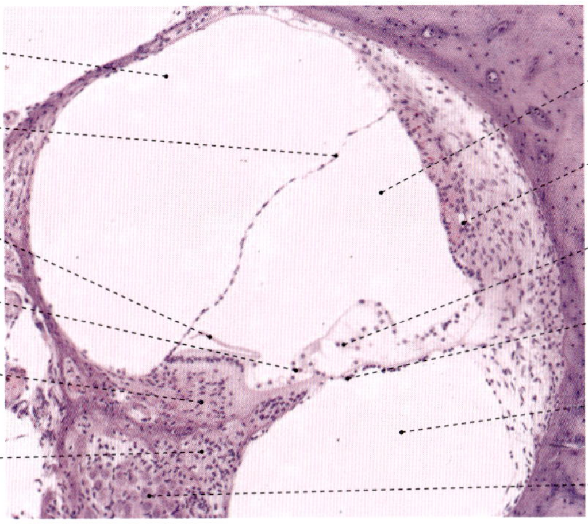

图 7-31 螺旋器（横断面）

Spiral organ. Transverse section

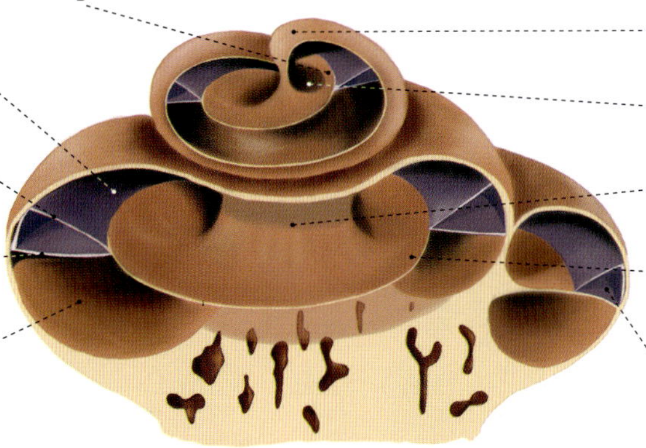

图 7-32 耳蜗模式图

Diagram of cochlea

第八章 内分泌腺

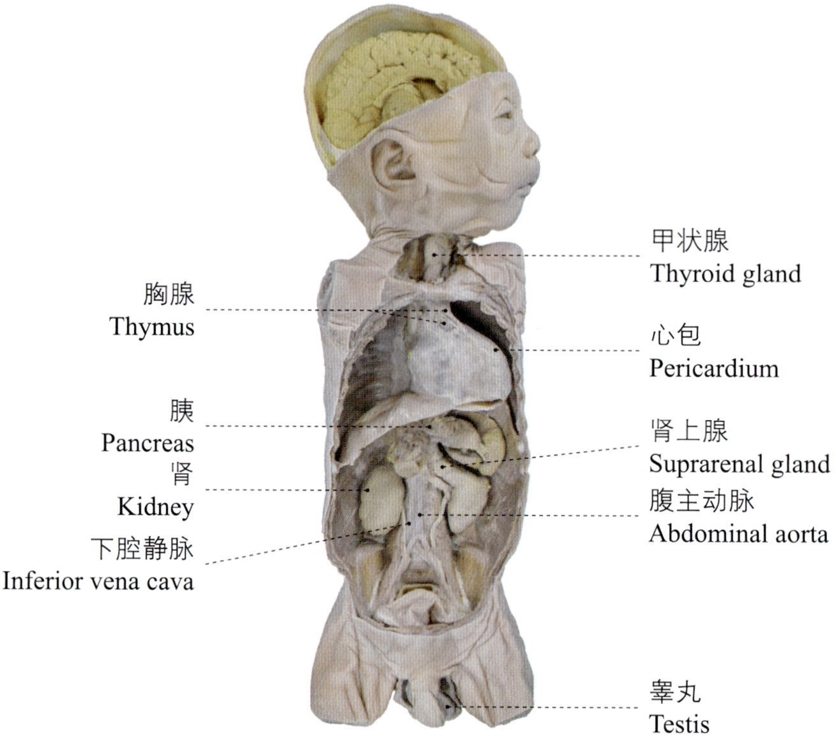

图 8–1 内分泌腺

Endocrine glands

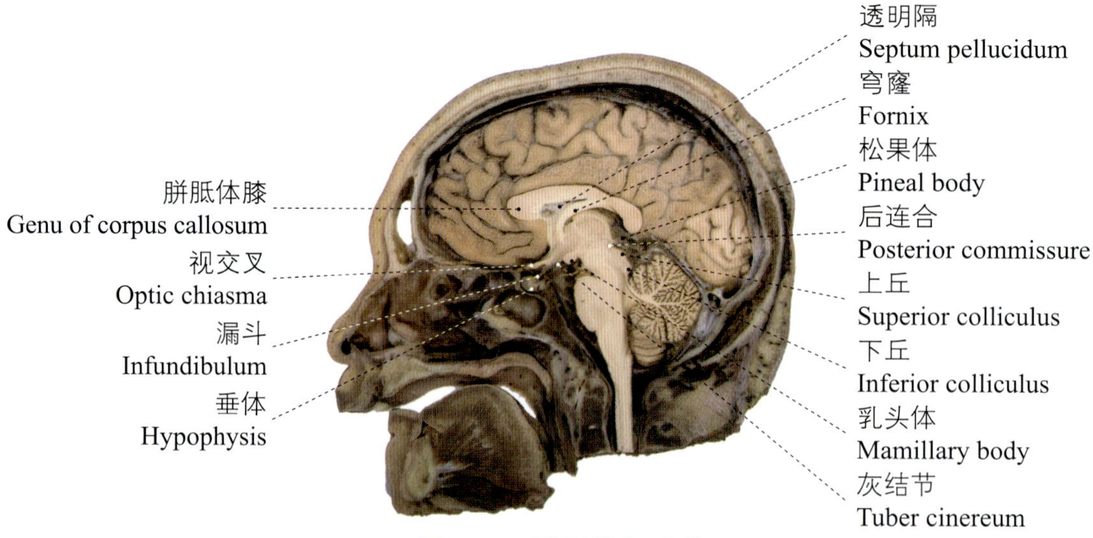

图 8–2 松果体和垂体

Pineal body and hypophysis

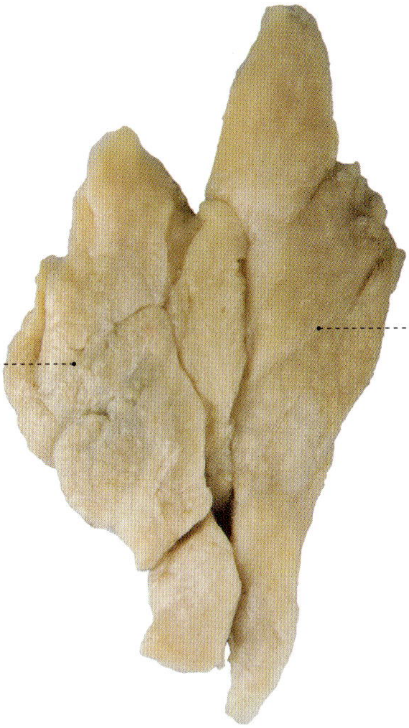

图 8-3　胸腺
Thymus

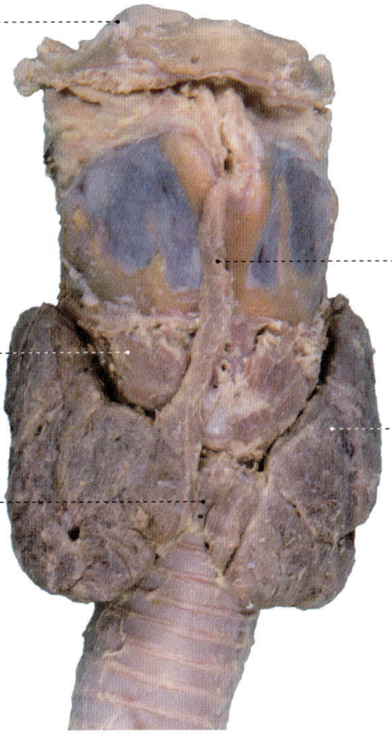

图 8-4　甲状腺（前面观）
Thyroid gland. Anterior aspect

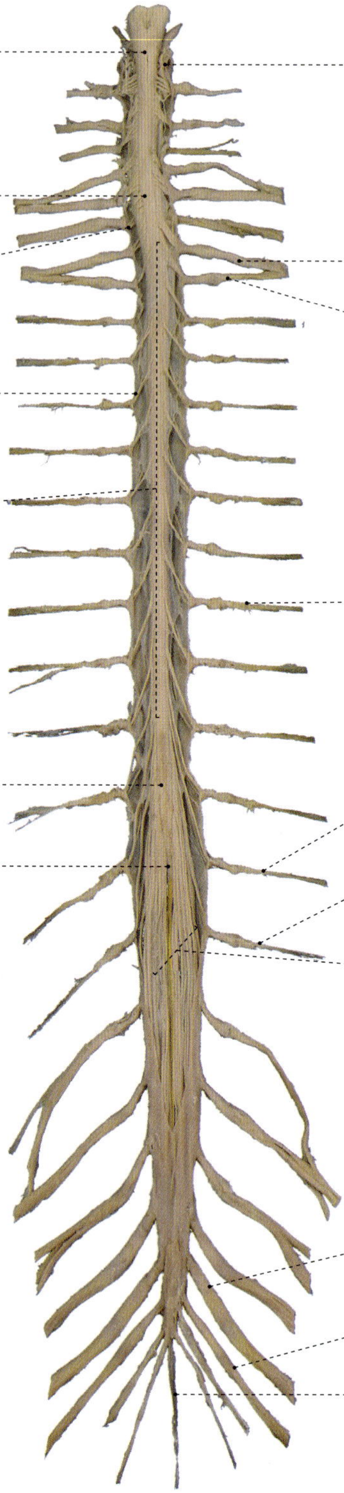

图 9–2　成人脊髓（后面观）

Spinal cord in adult. Posterior aspect

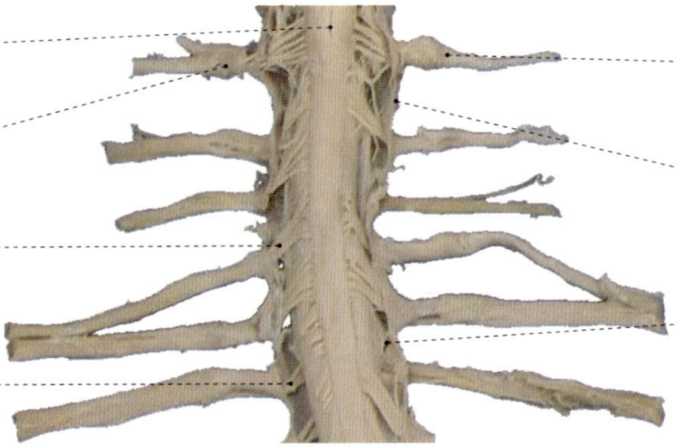

图 9–3　脊髓和脊神经根（后面观）

Spinal cord and roots of spinal nerves. Posterior aspect

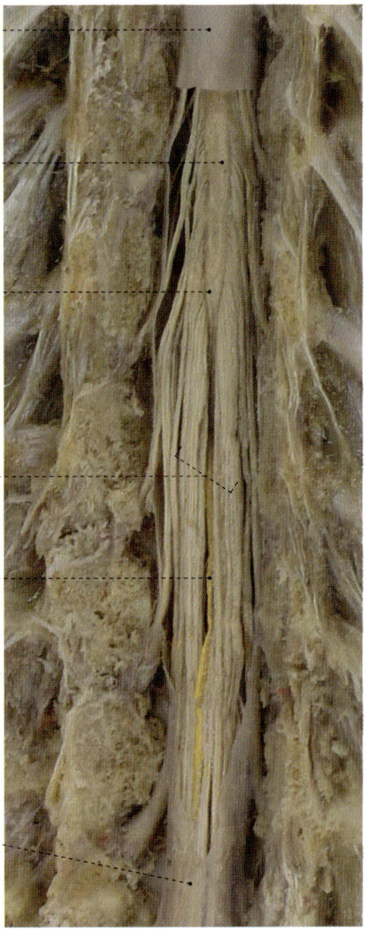

图 9–4　脊髓的被膜和脊神经根（后面观）

Meninges of spinal cord and roots of spinal nerves. Posterior aspect

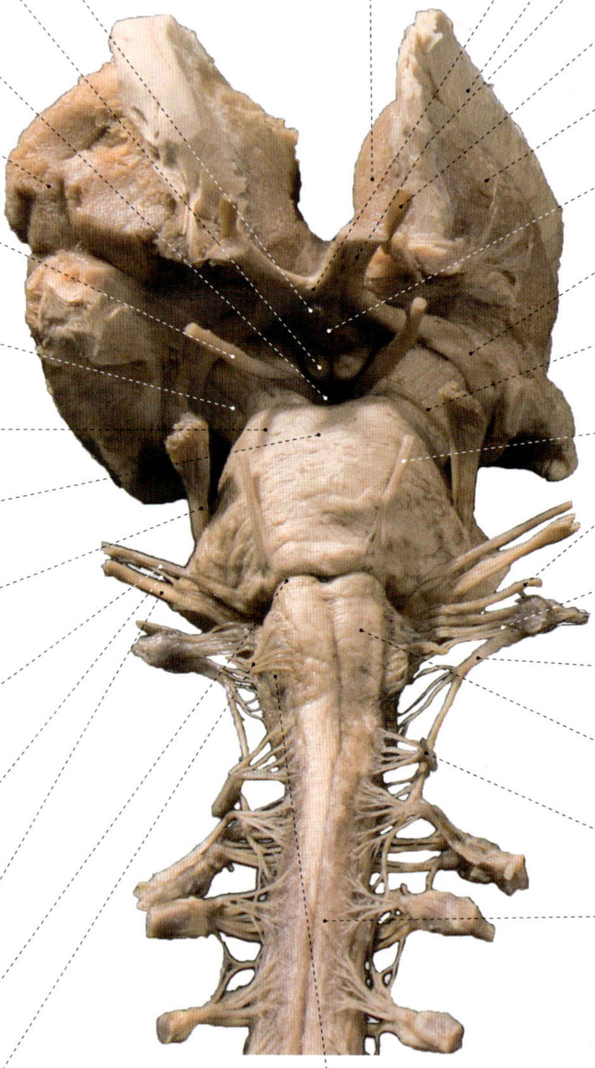

图 9-7　脑干（前面观）

Brain stem. Anterior aspect

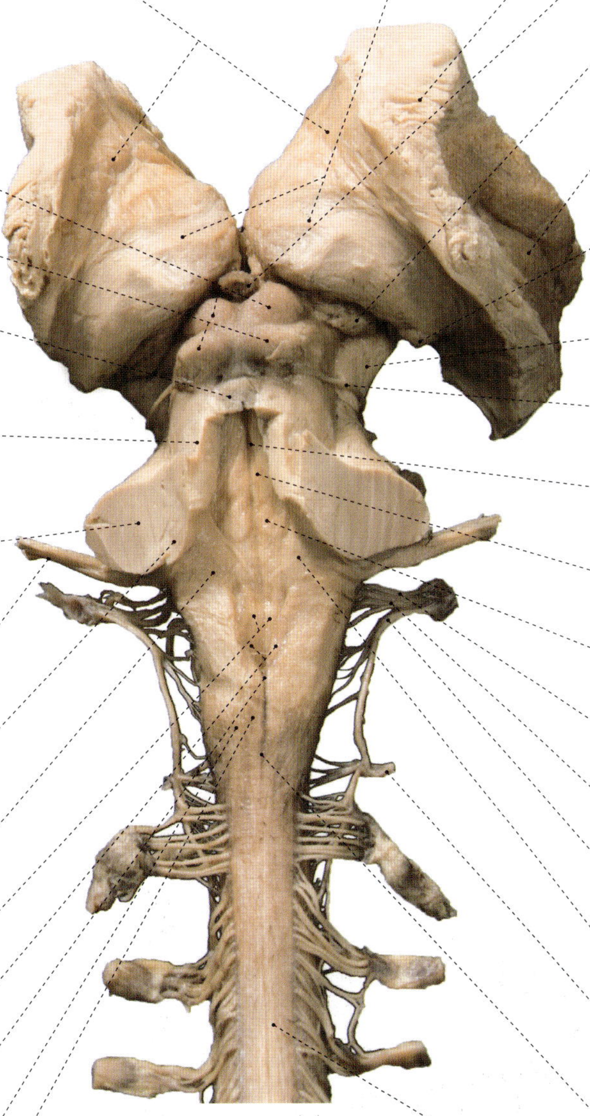

图 9–8　脑干（后面观）

Brain stem. Posterior aspect

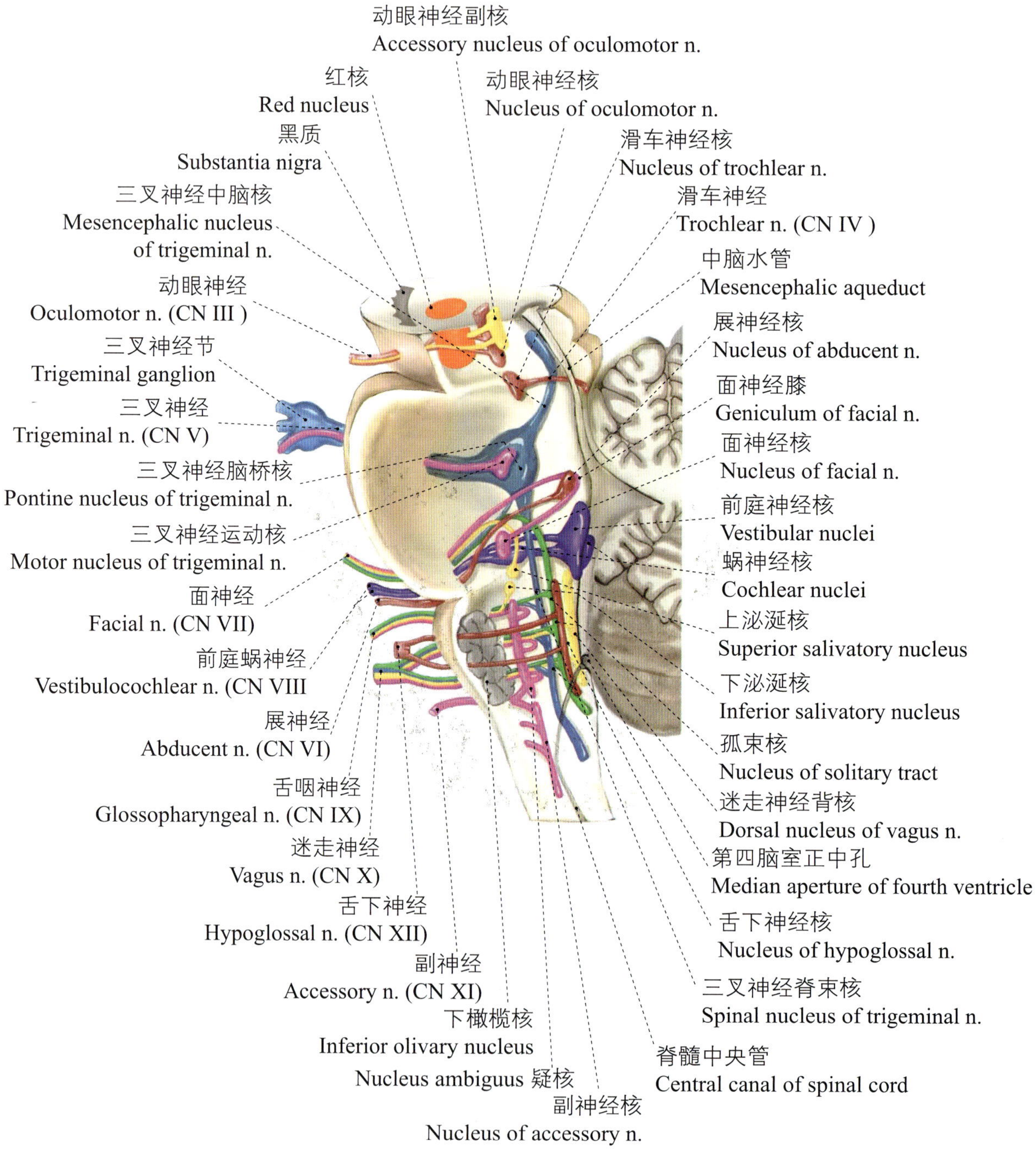

图 9–12　脑神经核模式图（内侧面观）

Diagram of nuclei of cranial n. Medial aspect

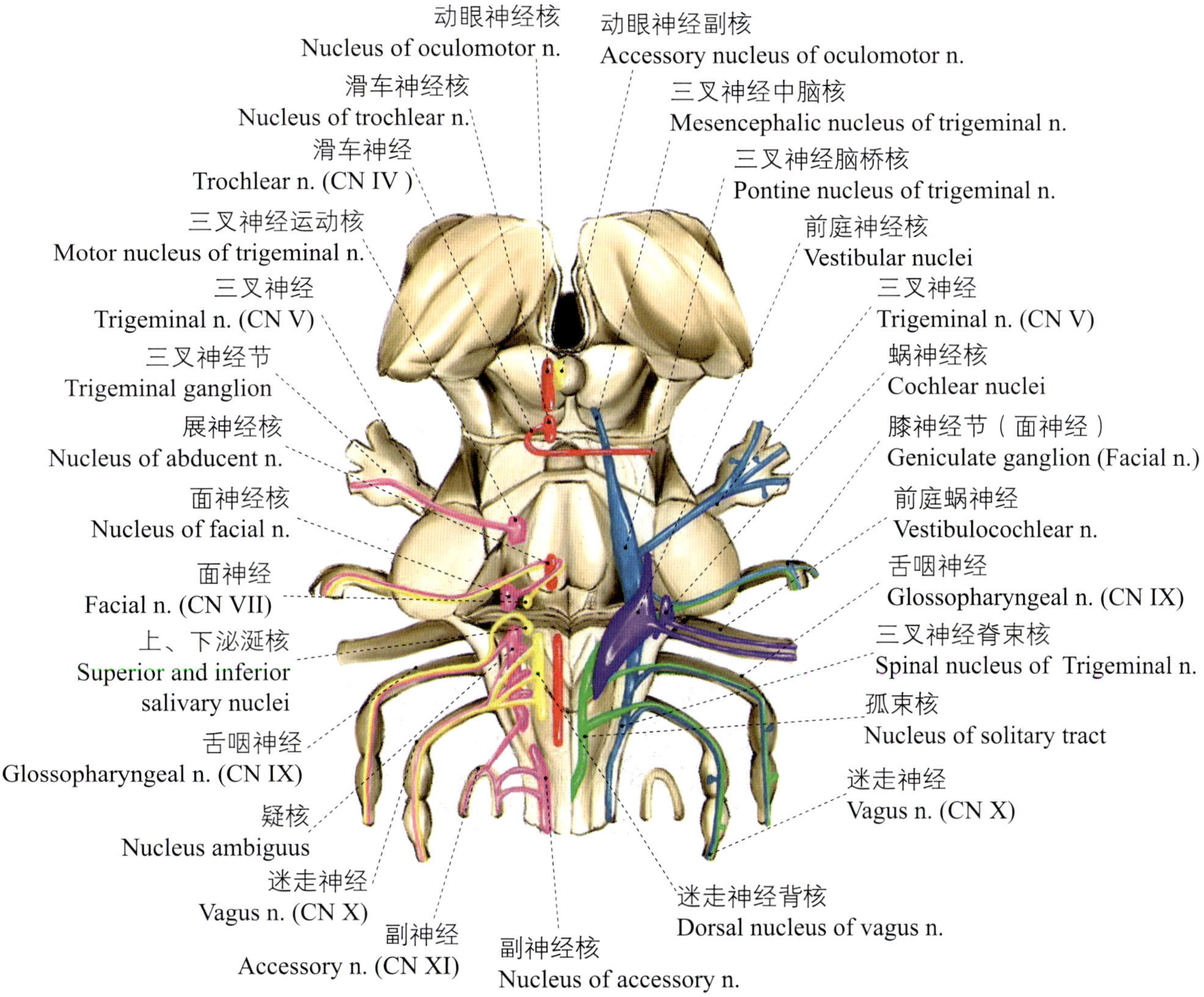

图 9–13　脑神经核模式图（后面观）

Diagram of nuclei of cranial n. Posterior aspect

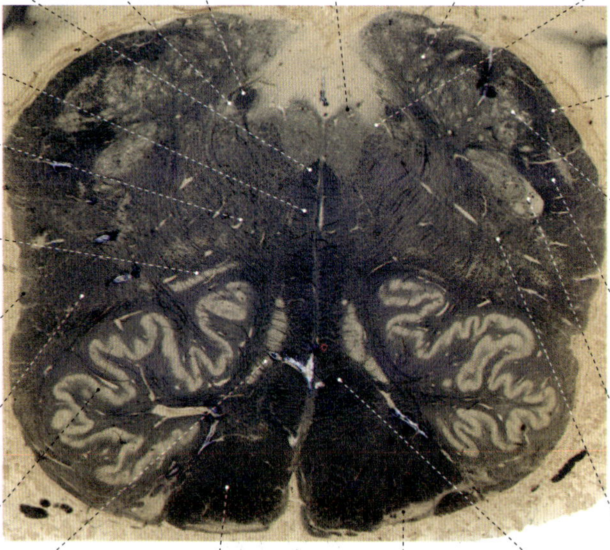

图 9–16　延髓横切面（经橄榄中部）

Transverse section of medulla oblongata through middle part of olive

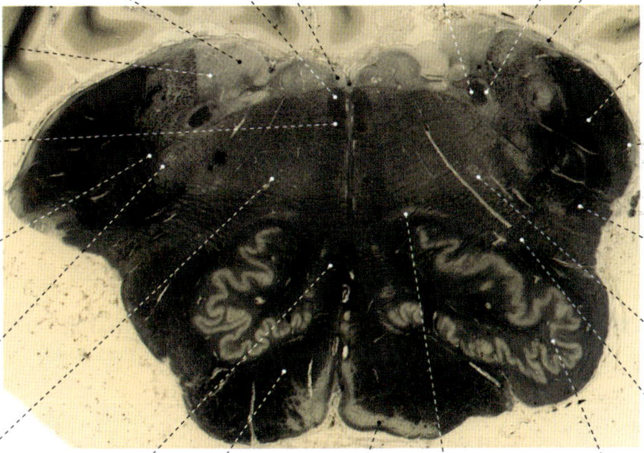

图 9–17　延髓横切面（经蜗神经核）

Transverse section of medulla oblongata through cochlear nuclei

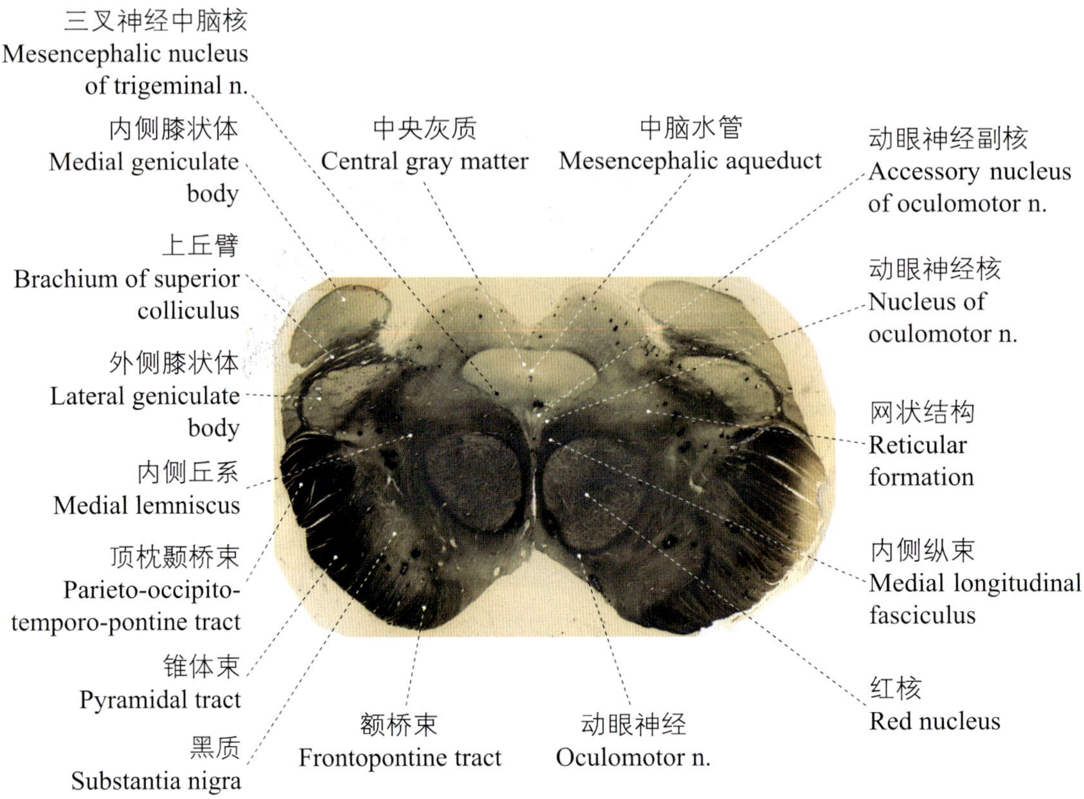

图 9-21　中脑横切面（经上丘）

Transverse section of midbrain through superior colliculus

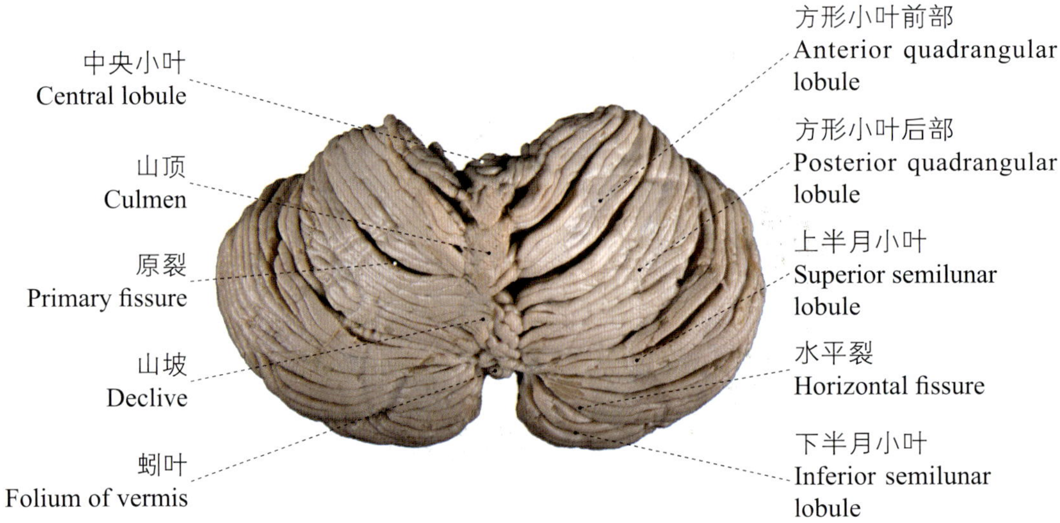

图 9-22　小脑（上面观）

Cerebellum. Superior aspect

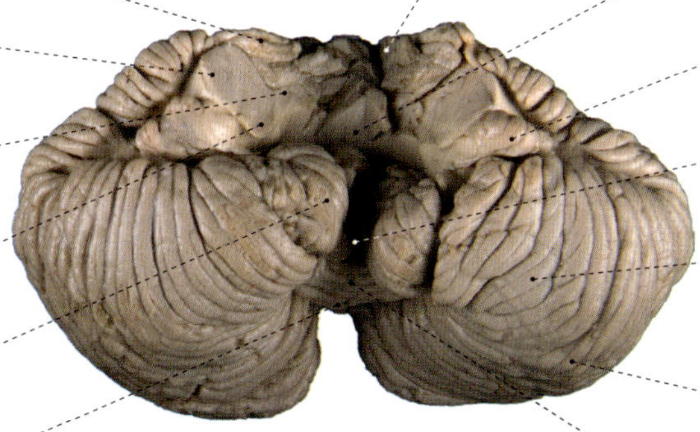

图 9–23　小脑（下面观）

Cerebellum. Inferior aspect

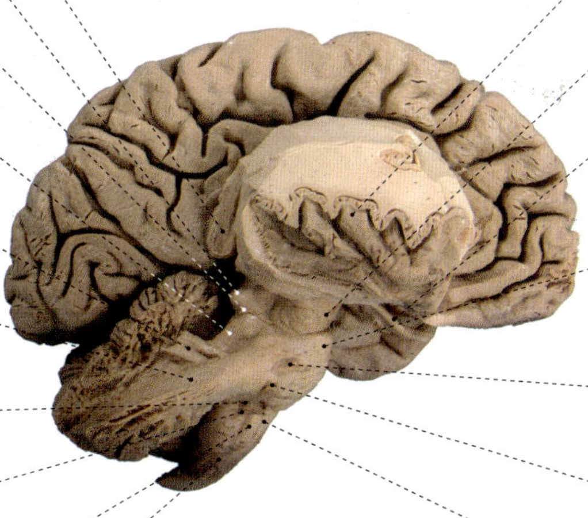

图 9–24　小脑脚

Cerebellar peduncles

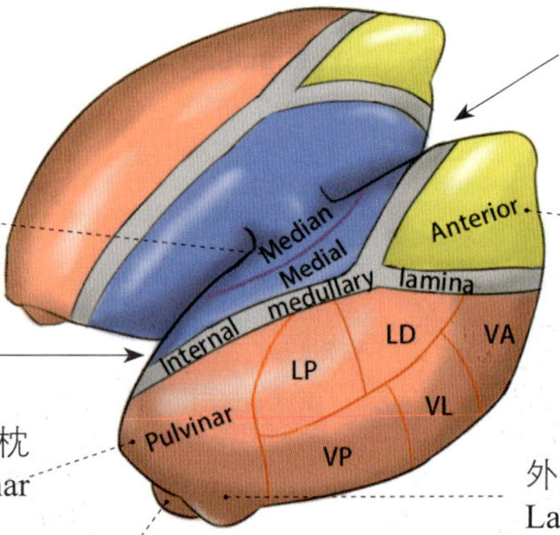

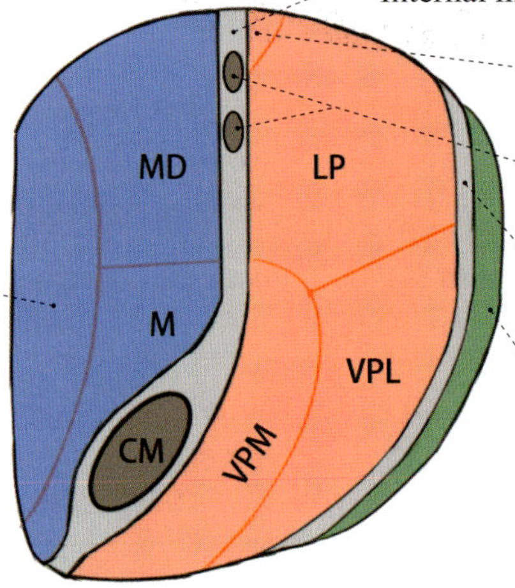

Thalamic nuclei 丘脑核

CM Centromedian nucleus 中央中核
LP Lateral posterior nucleus 后外侧核
MD Medial dorsal 背内侧核
VL Ventral lateral nucleus 腹外侧核
VPM Ventral posteromedial nucleus 腹后内侧核
LD Lateral dorsal nucleus 背外侧核
M Medial nuclear group 内侧核群
VA Ventral anterior nucleus 腹前核
VP Ventral posterior nuclei 腹后核
VPL Ventral posterolateral 腹后外侧核

经腹后核的丘脑冠状断面示意图（后面观）
Diagram of coronal section of thalamus through ventral posterior nuclei. Posterior aspect

图 9-28 丘脑核团模式图

Diagram of thalamic nuclei

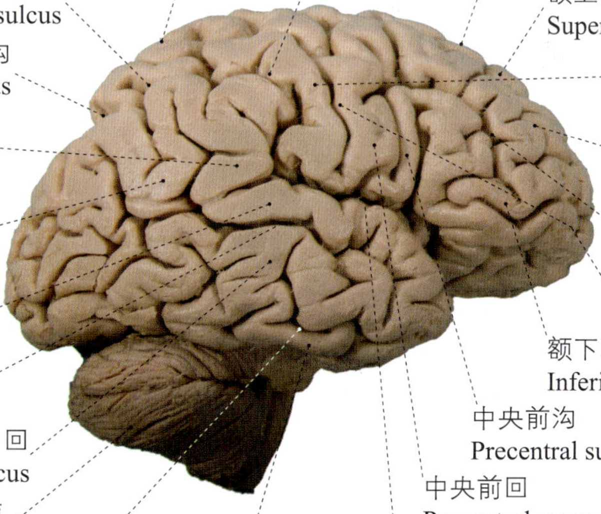

图 9–29 脑（外侧面观）

Brain. Lateral aspect

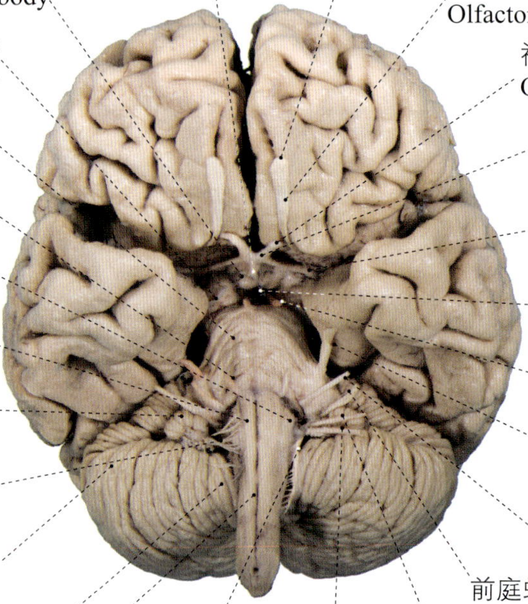

图 9–30　脑（底面观）

Brain. Basal aspect

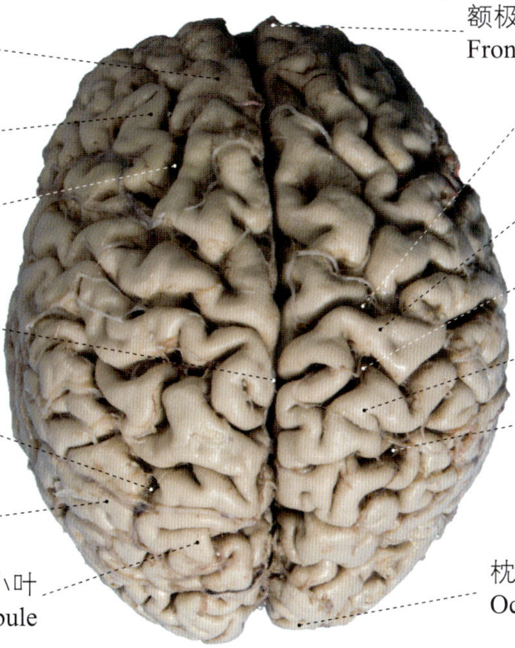

图 9-31 脑（上面观）
Brain. Superior aspect

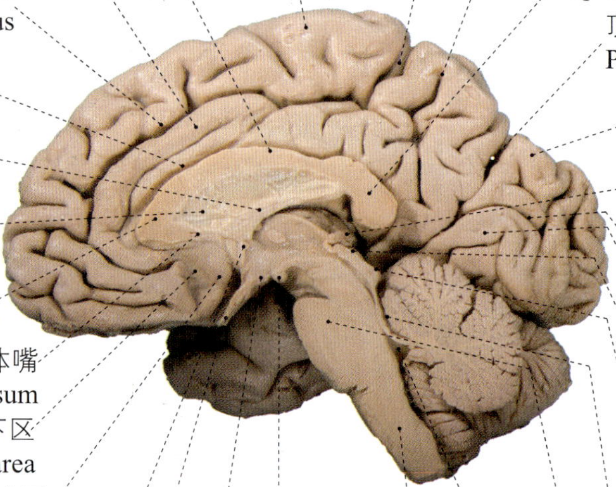

图 9–32　脑（正中矢状切面）（1）

Brain. Median saggital section (1)

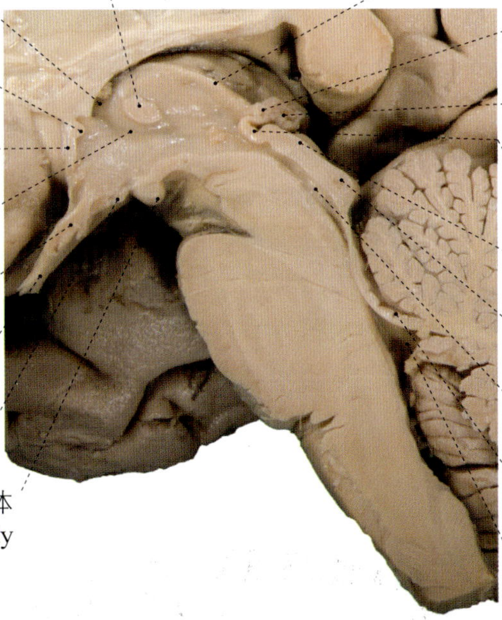

图 9–33　脑（正中矢状切面）（2）

Brain. Median saggital section (2)

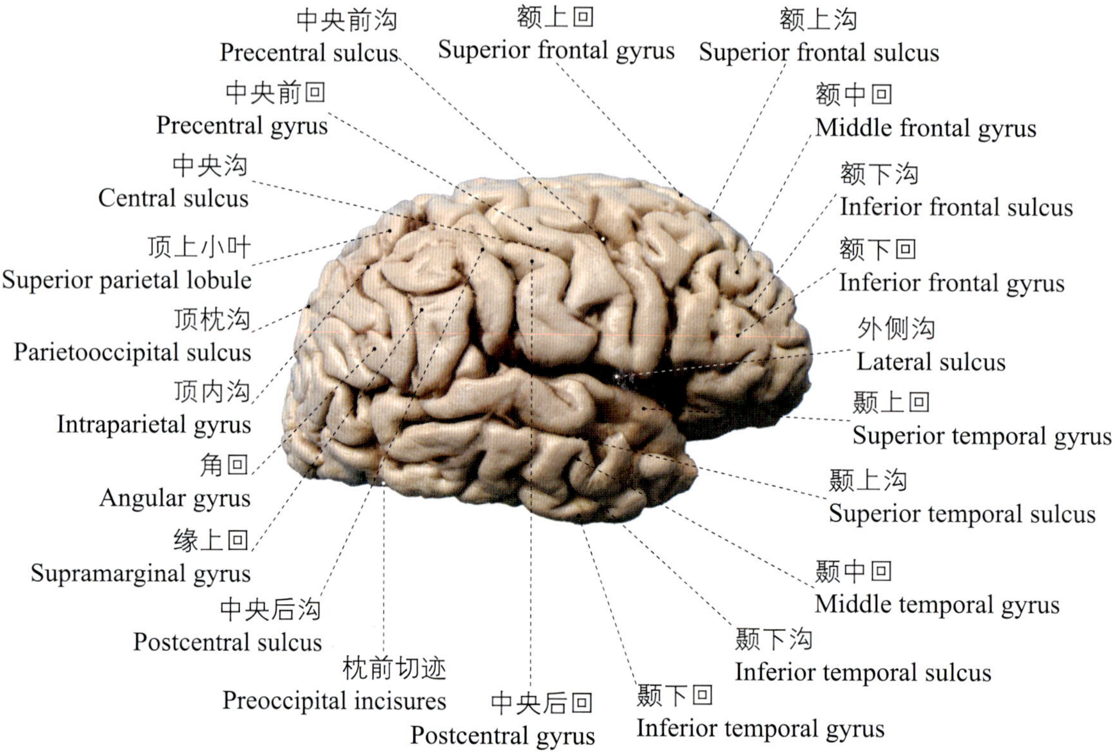

图 9–34　大脑半球（外侧面观）

Cerebral hemisphere. Lateral aspect

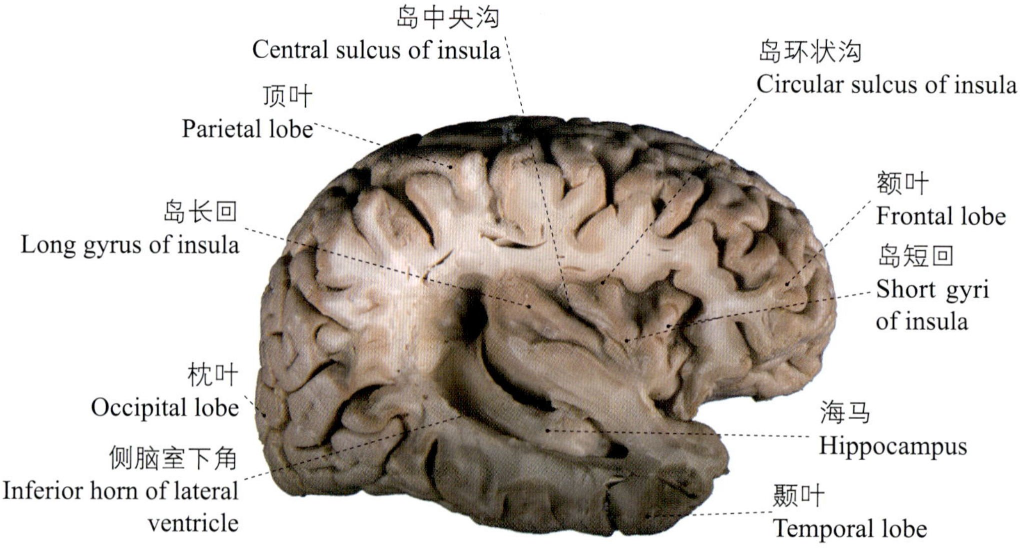

图 9–35　岛叶

Insular lobe

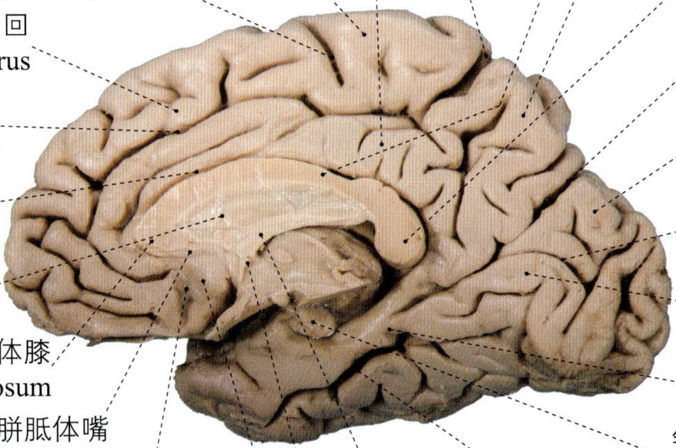

图 9–36　大脑半球（内侧面观）

Cerebral hemisphere. Medial aspect

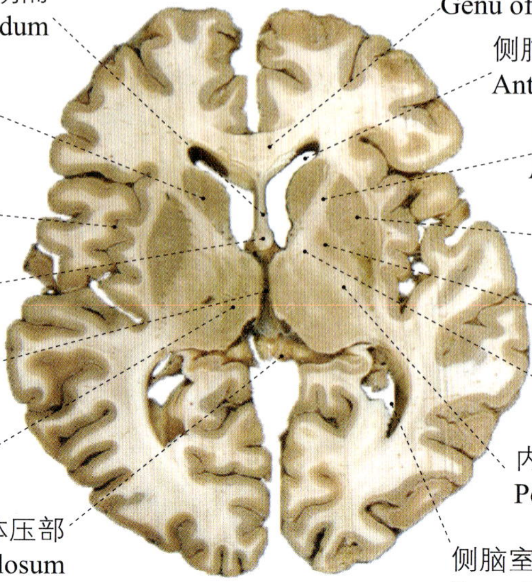

图 9–37　脑的水平切面

Horizontal section of brain

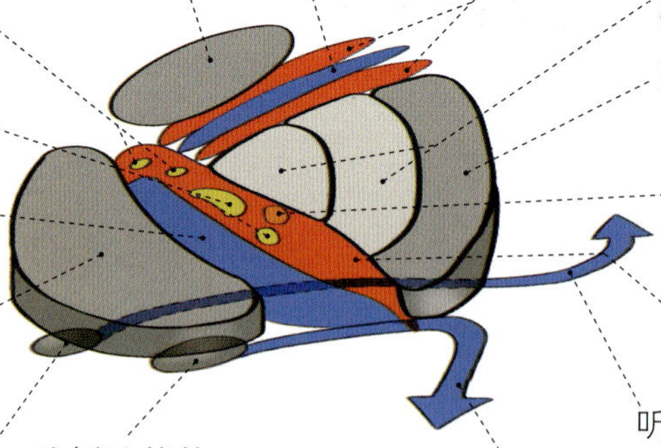

图 9–38　内囊模式图

Diagram of Internal capsule

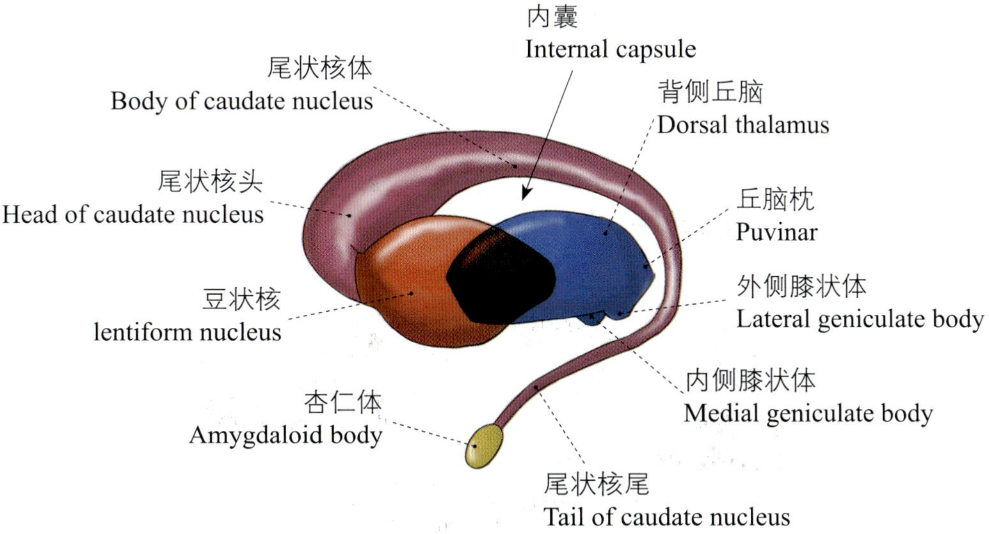

图 9–39　基底核模式图

Diagram of basal nuclei

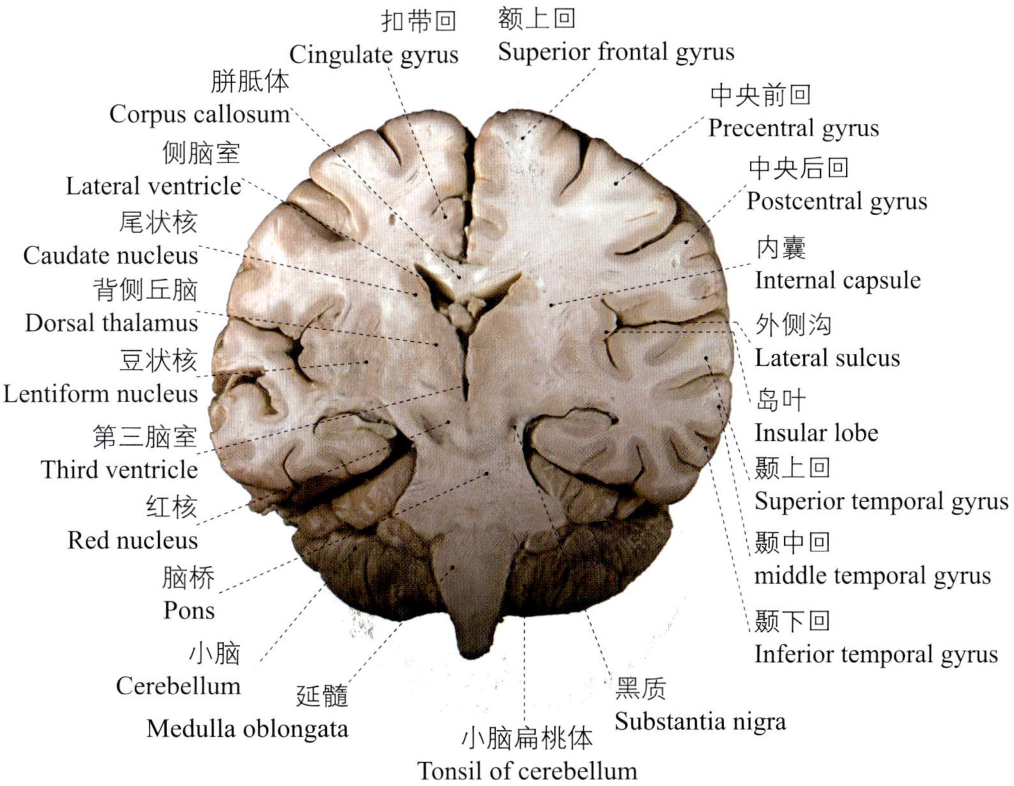

图 9–40　脑的冠状切面

Coronal section of brain

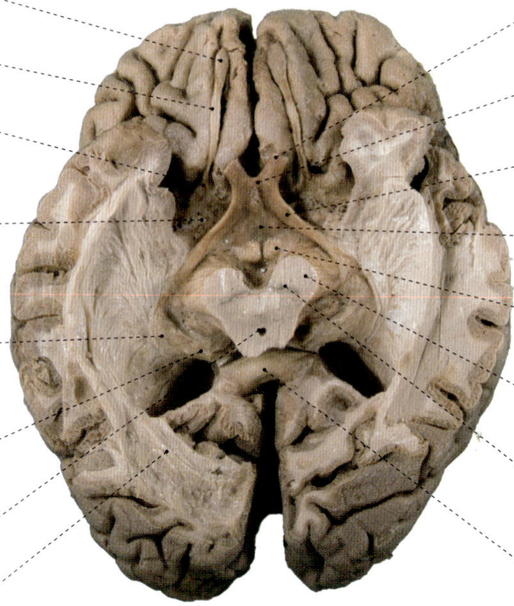

图 9–45　视束及视辐射

Optic tract and optic radiation

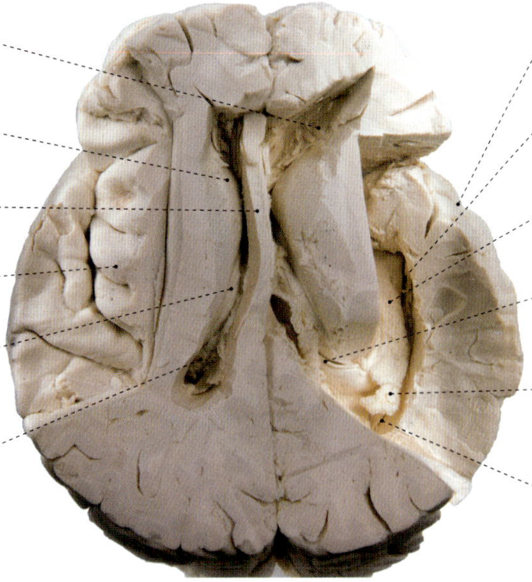

图 9–46　侧脑室（上面观）

Lateral ventricle. Superior aspect

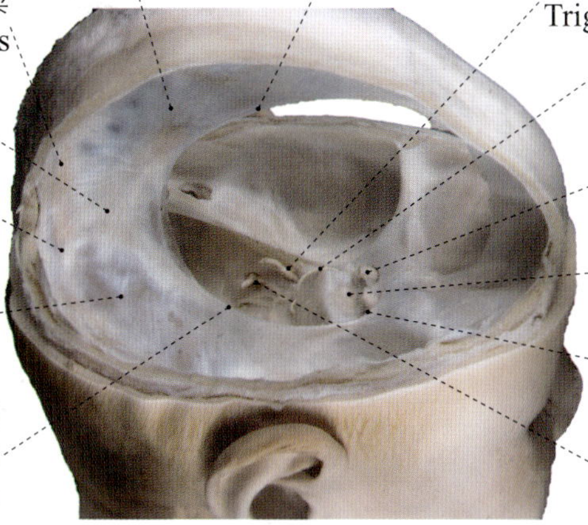

图 9–47　硬脑膜

Cerebral dura mater

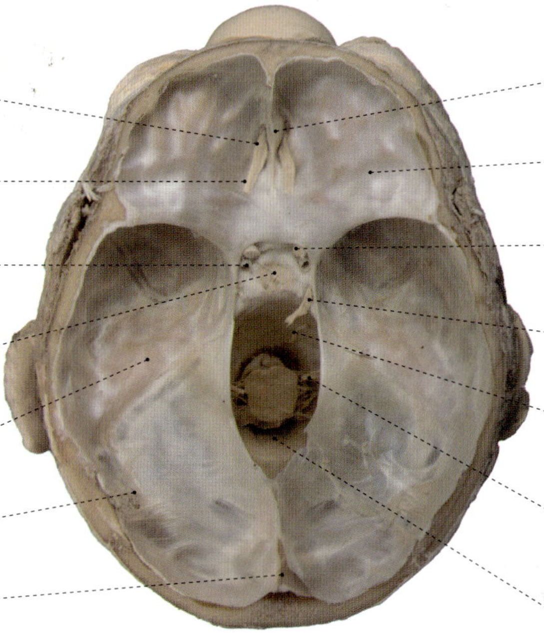

图 9–48　颅底的硬脑膜

Dura mater of base of skull

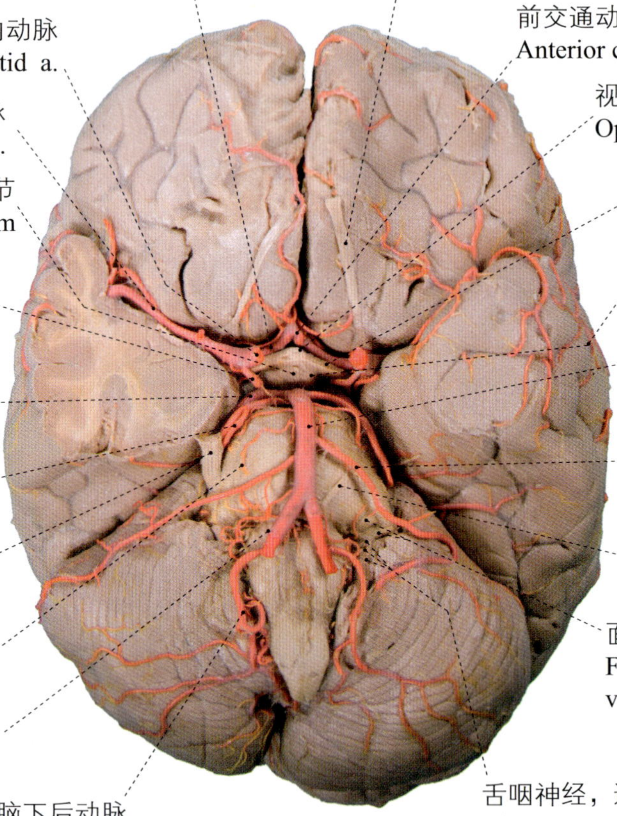

图 9–49　脑底的动脉

Arteries at base of brain

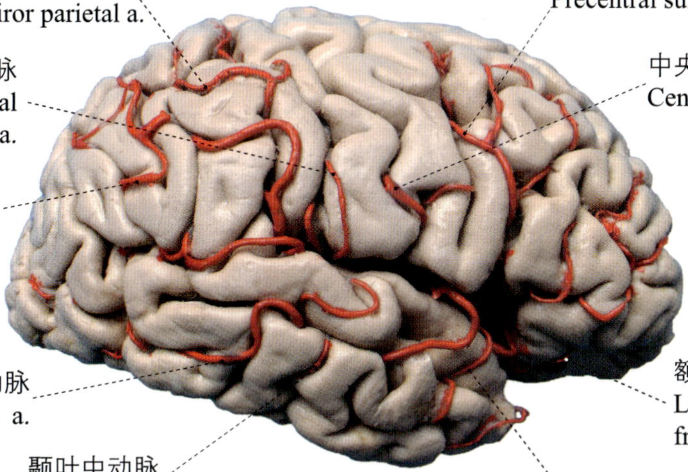

图 9-50 大脑半球外侧面动脉

Arteries of lateral surface of cerebral hemisphere

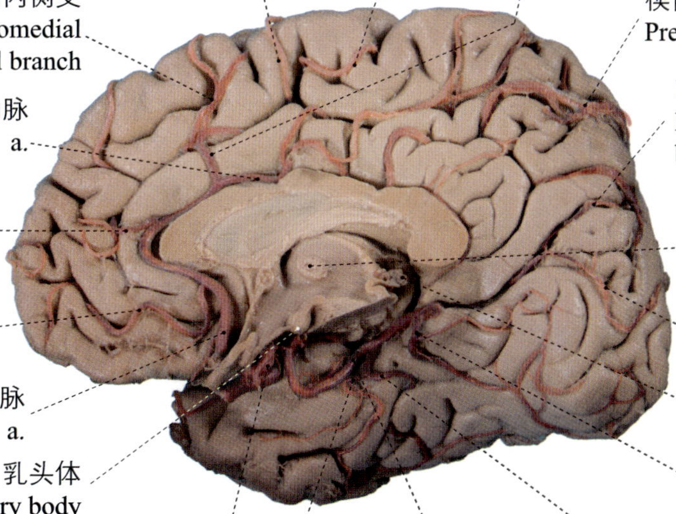

图 9-51 大脑半球内侧面动脉

Arteries of medial surface of cerebral hemisphere

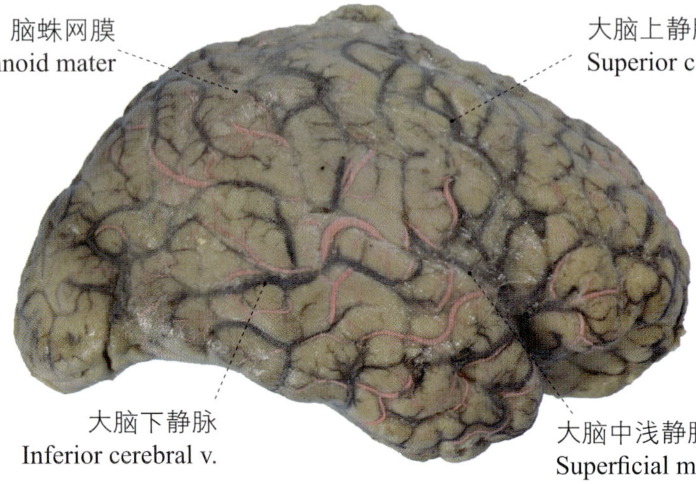

图 9–52 大脑半球外侧面血管

Blood vessels of lateral surface of cerebral hemisphere

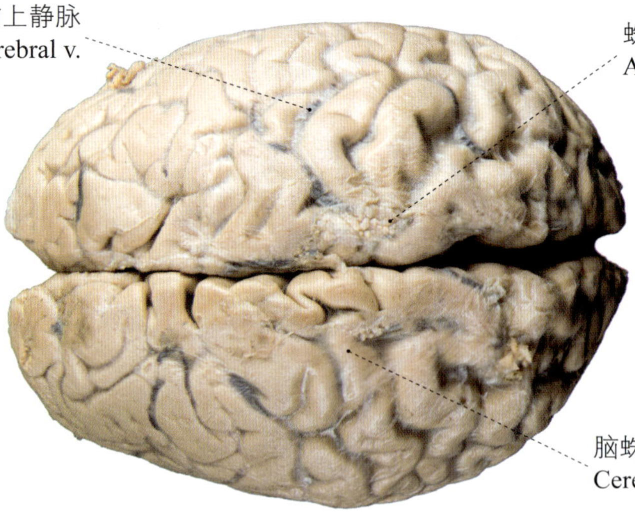

图 9–53 脑蛛网膜

Cerebral arachnoid mater

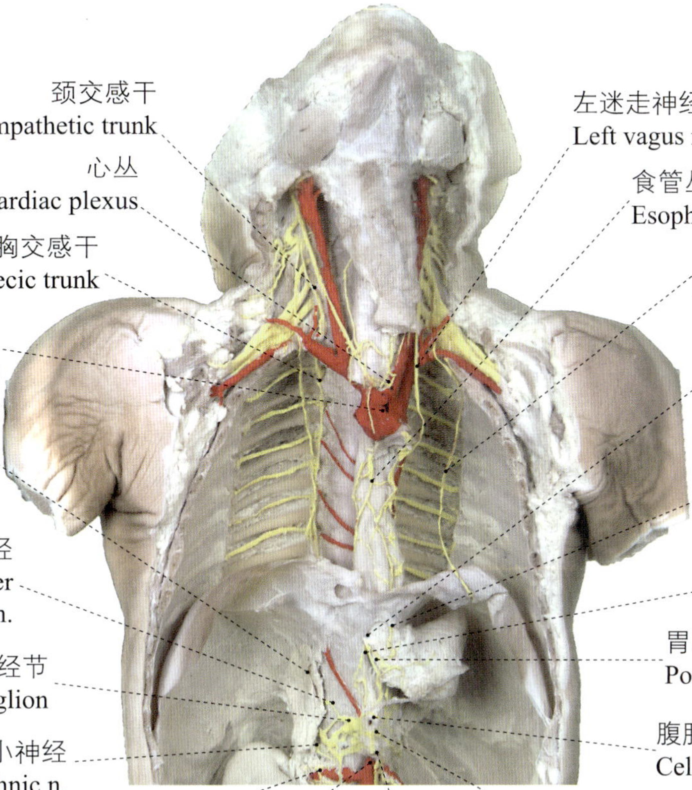

图 9–54 内脏神经（前面观）（1）

Visceral nerves. Anterior aspect (1)

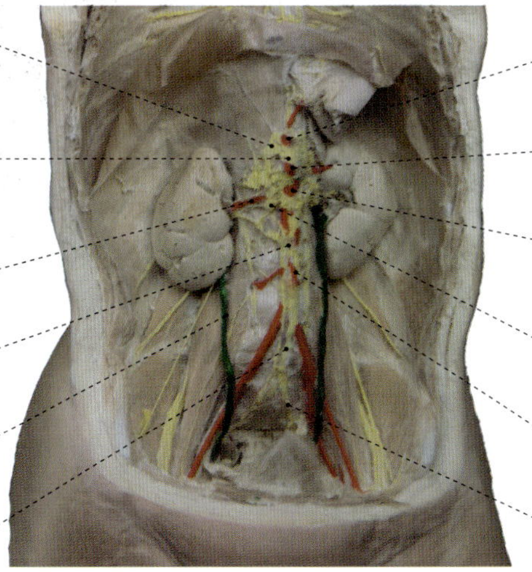

图 9–55 内脏神经（前面观）（2）

Visceral nerves. Anterior aspect (2)

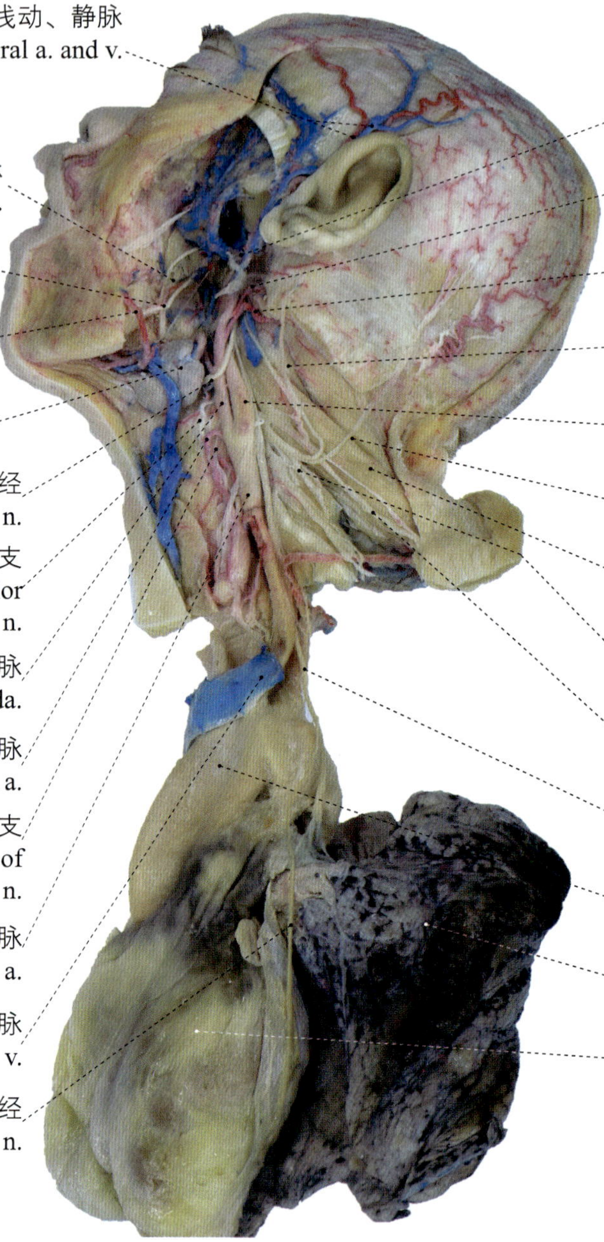

图 9–56　迷走神经和副神经（左侧面观）

Left vagus n. and accessory n. Left aspect

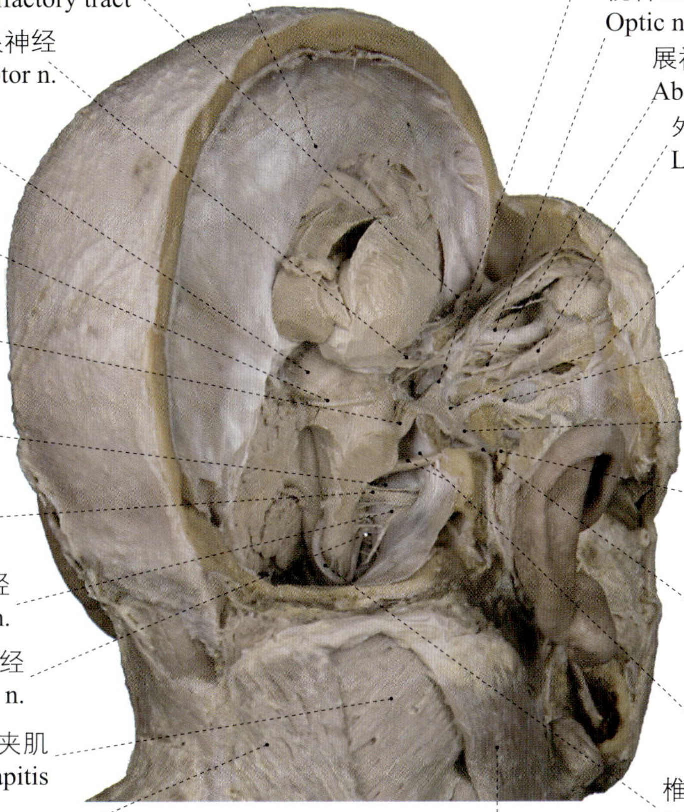

图 9–57　脑神经（后上面观）
Cranial nerves. Posterosuperior aspect

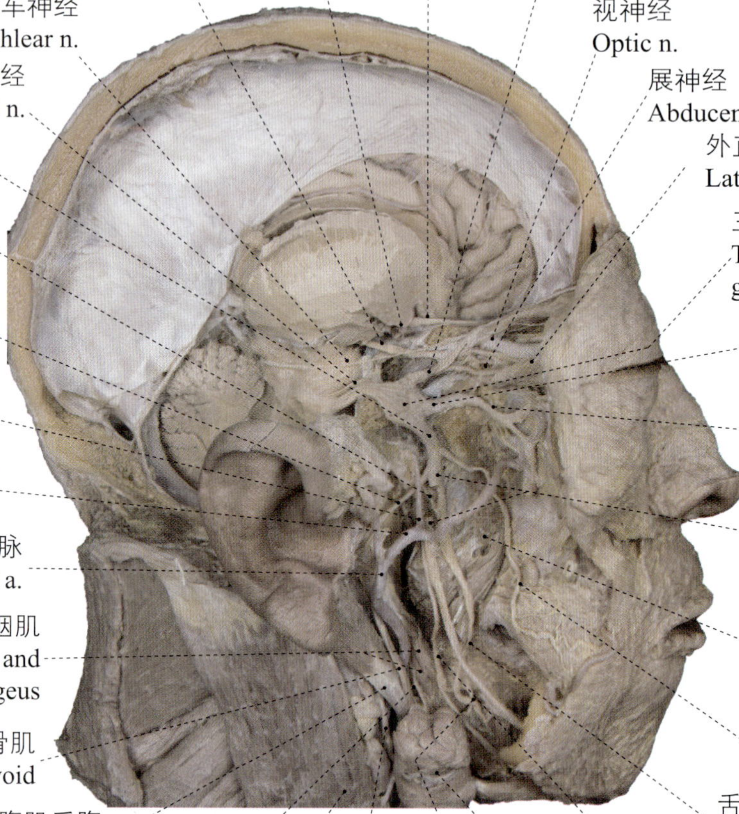

图 9–58　脑神经（外侧面）

Cranial nerves. Lateral aspect

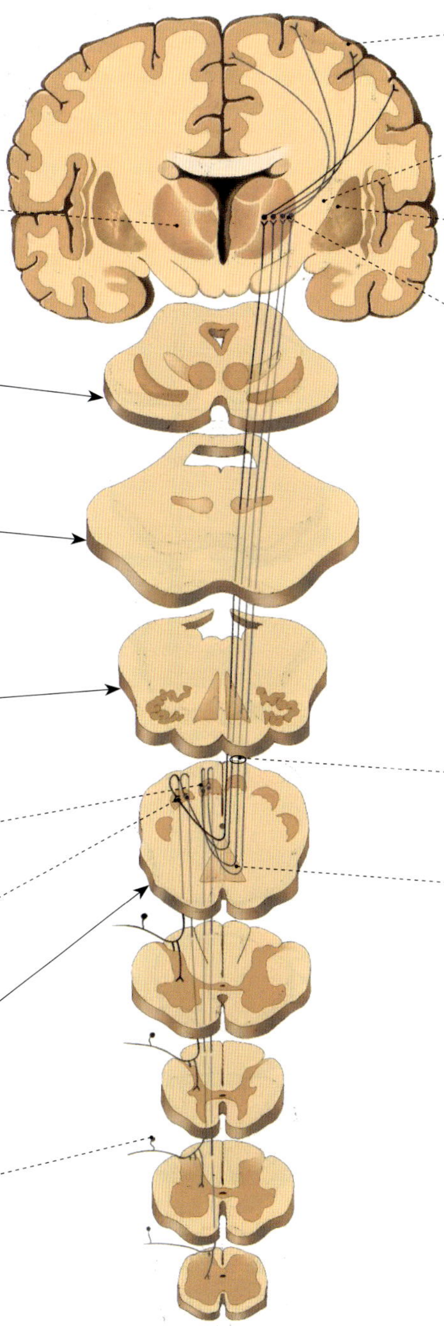

图 9–59 意识性本体感觉传导路（躯干和四肢）

Conscious proprioceptive pathway. Trunk and limbs

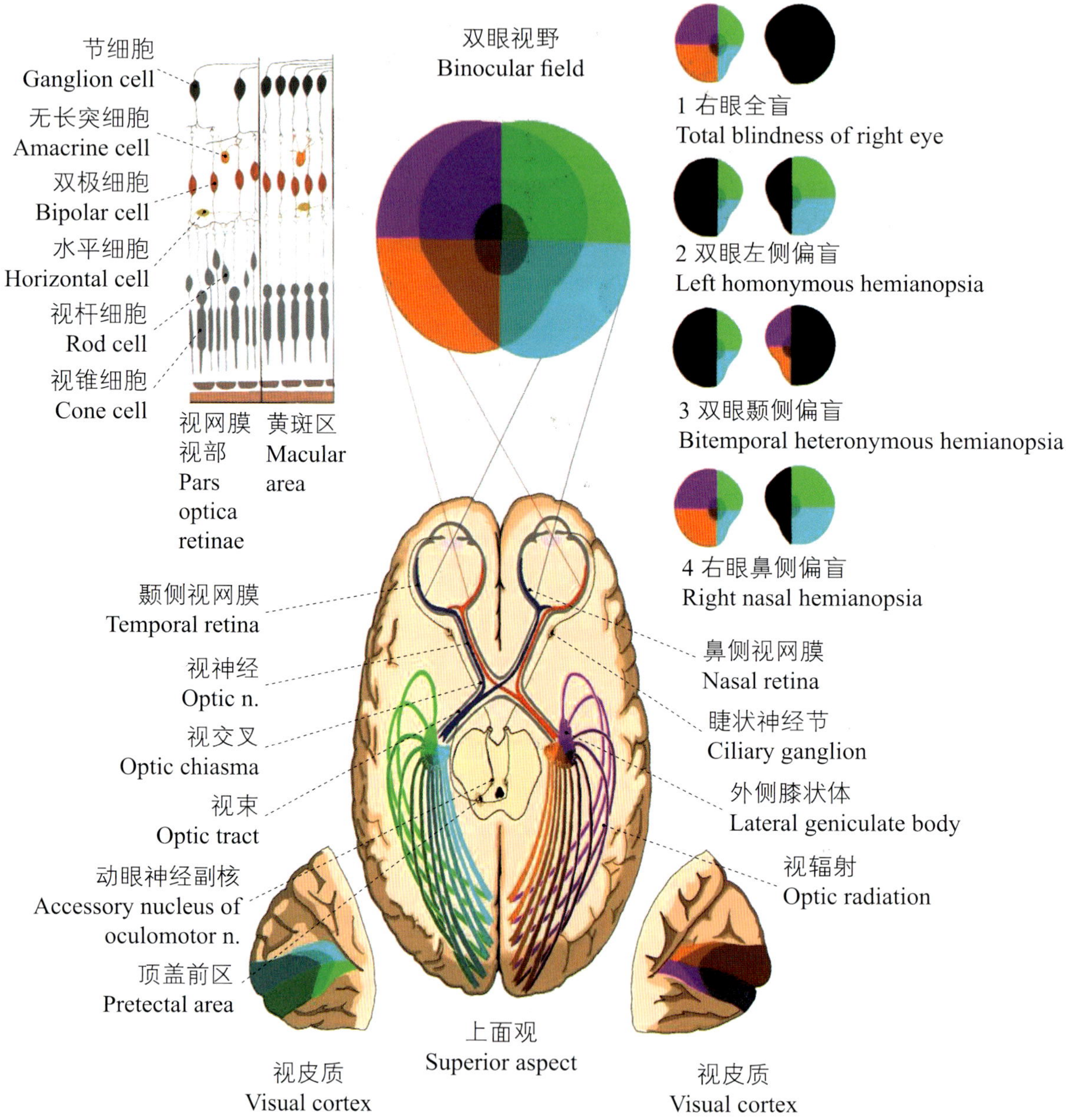

图 9–62　视觉传导路

Visual pathway

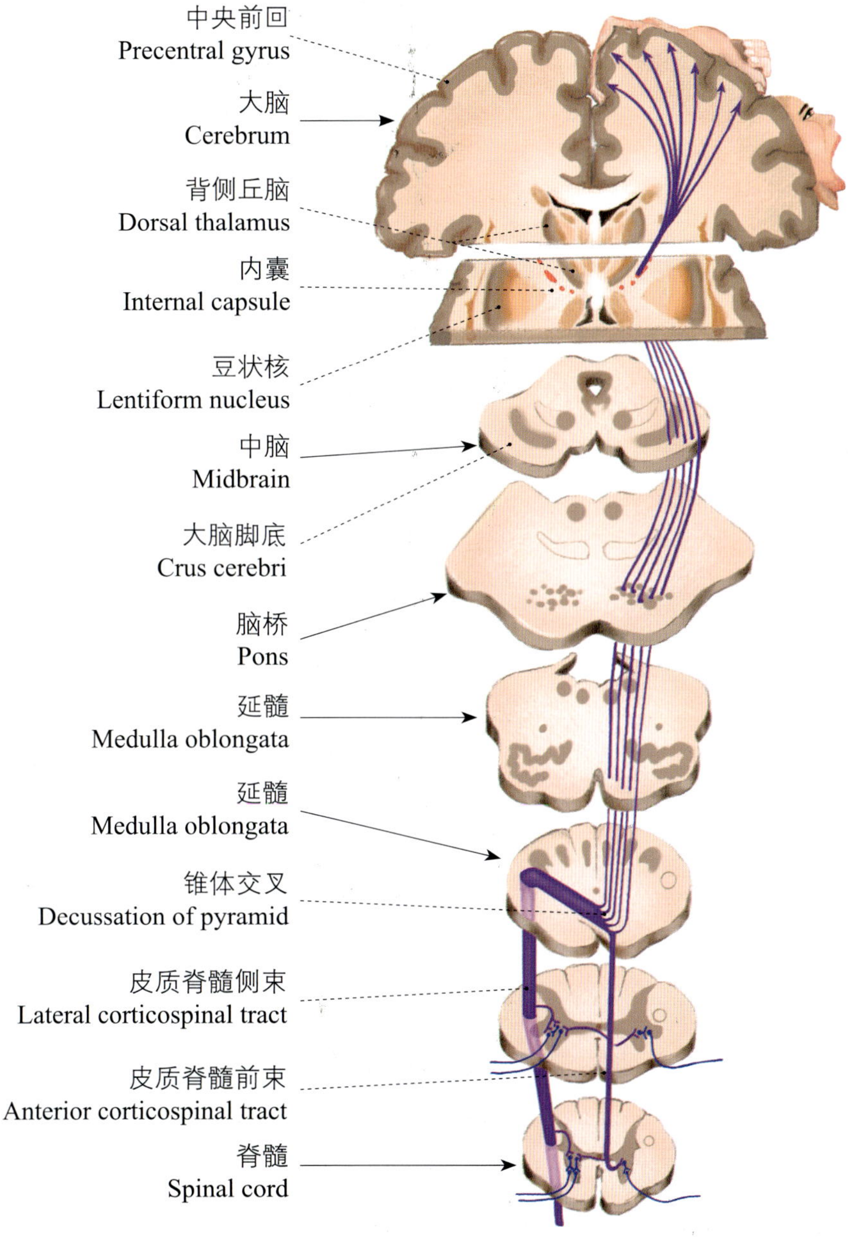

图 9–63 锥体系（皮质脊髓束）

Pyramidal system. Corticospinal tract

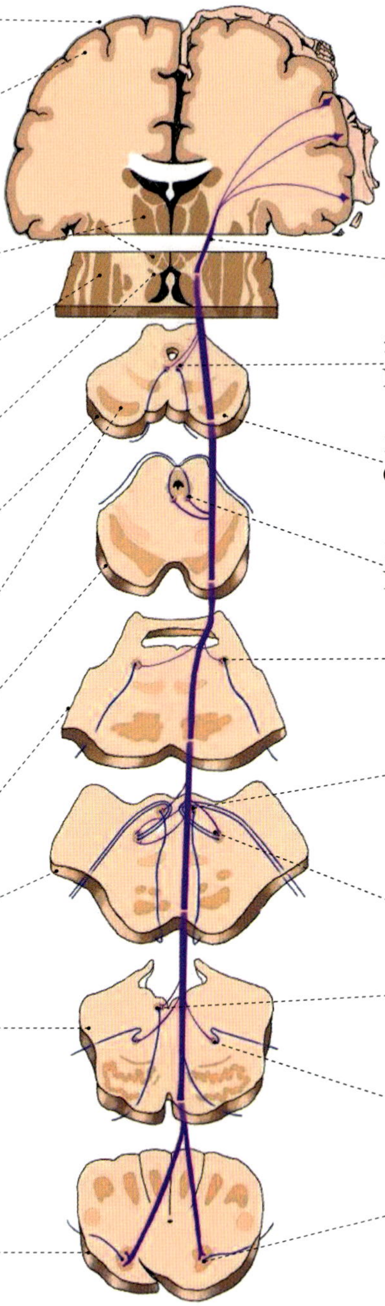

图 9–64 锥体系（皮质核束）

Pyramidal system. Corticonuclear tract

第十章　局部解剖

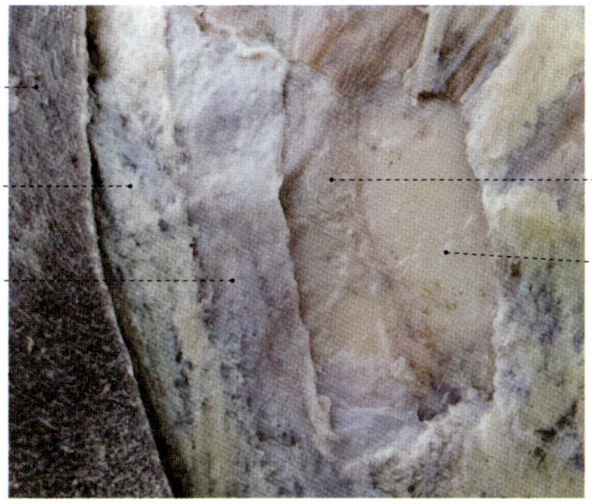

图 10–1　头皮层次

Layers of scalp

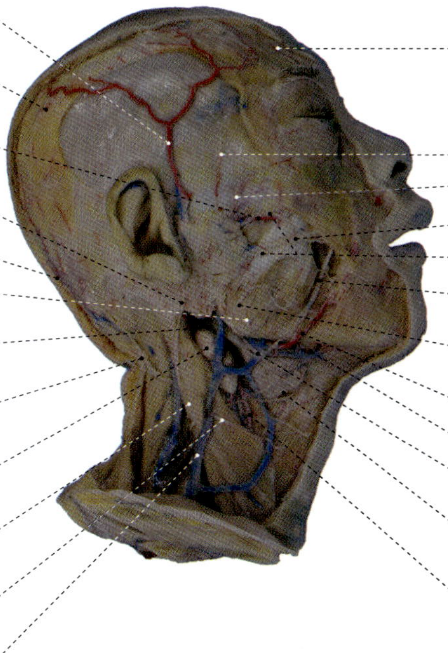

图 10–2　头面颈部的肌肉、血管和神经（外侧面观）（1）

Muscles, blood vessels and nerves of head, face and neck. Lateral aspect (1)

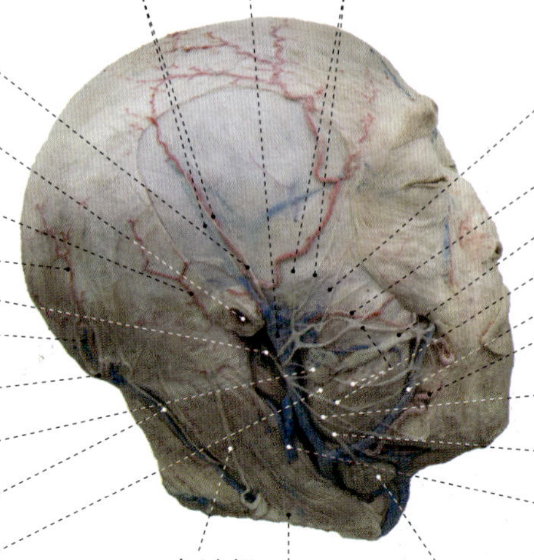

图 10–3　头颈部的肌肉、血管和神经（外侧面观）（2）

Muscles, blood vessels and nerves of head and neck. Lateral aspect (2)

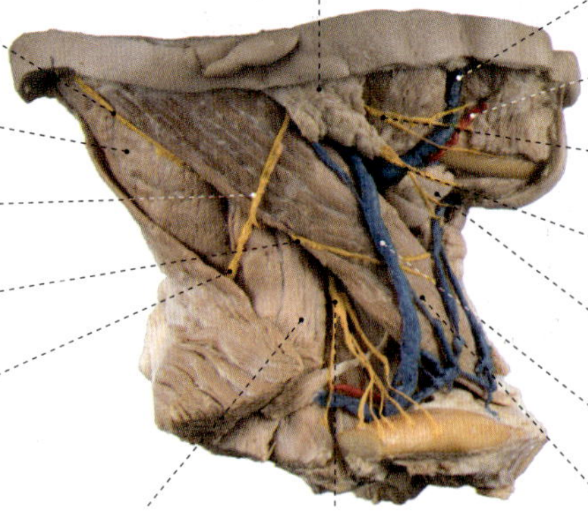

图 10–4　头颈部的肌肉、血管和神经（外侧面观）（3）

Muscles, blood vessels and nerves of head and neck. Lateral aspect (3)

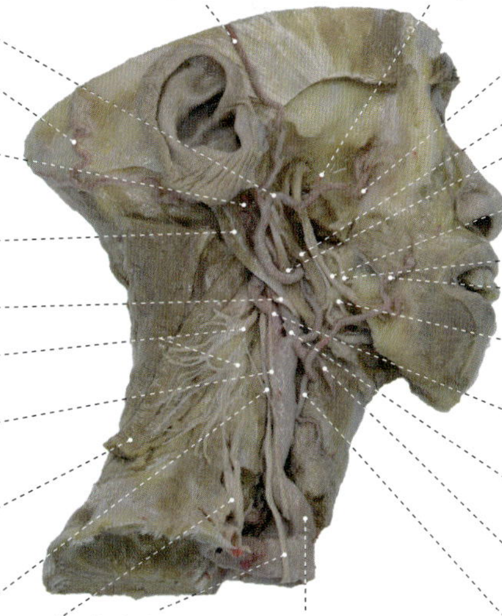

图 10–5 头颈部的肌肉、血管和神经（外侧面观）（4）

Muscles, blood vessels and nerves of head and neck. Lateral aspect (4)

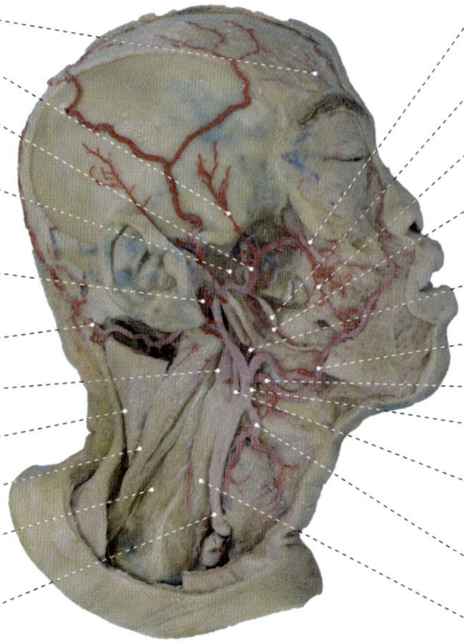

图 10–6 头颈部的肌肉、血管和神经（外侧面观）（5）

Muscles, blood vessels and nerves of head and neck. Lateral aspect (5)

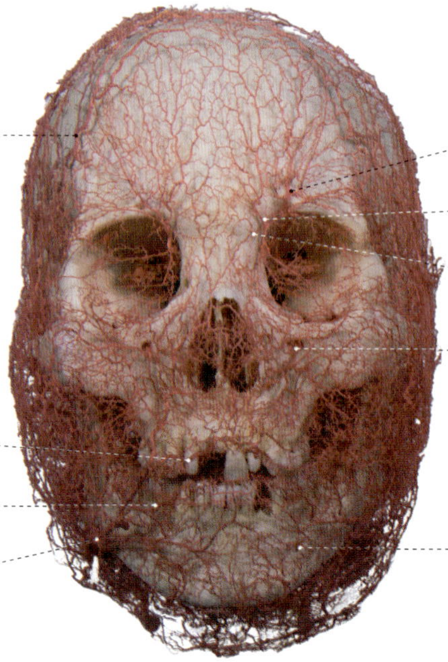

图 10–11　头部的动脉铸型（前面观）

Cast of arteries of head. Anterior aspect

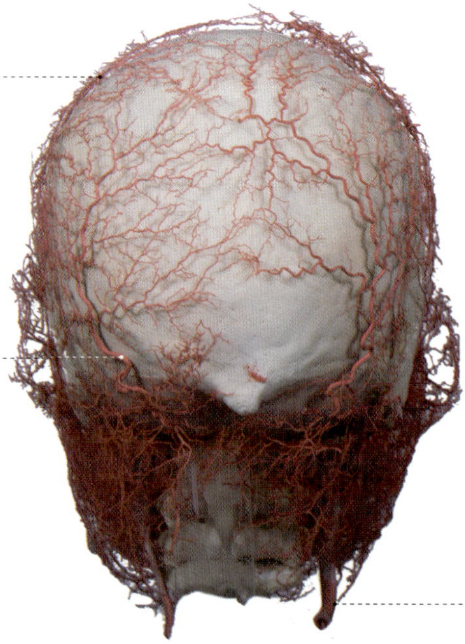

图 10–12　头部的动脉铸型（后面观）

Cast of arteries of head. Posterior aspect

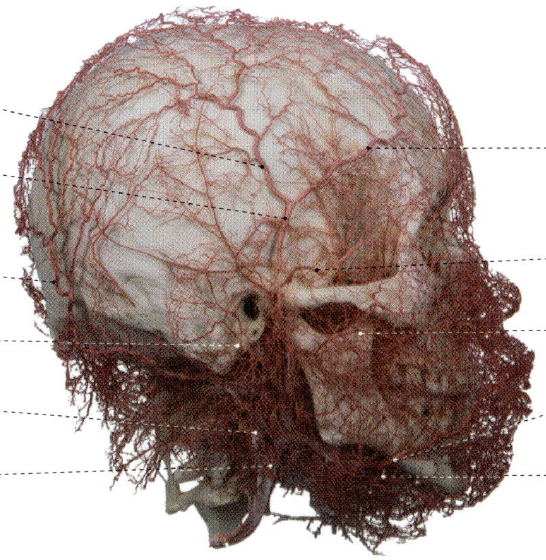

图 10–13　头部的动脉铸型（外侧面观）（1）
Cast of arteries of the head. Lateral aspect (1)

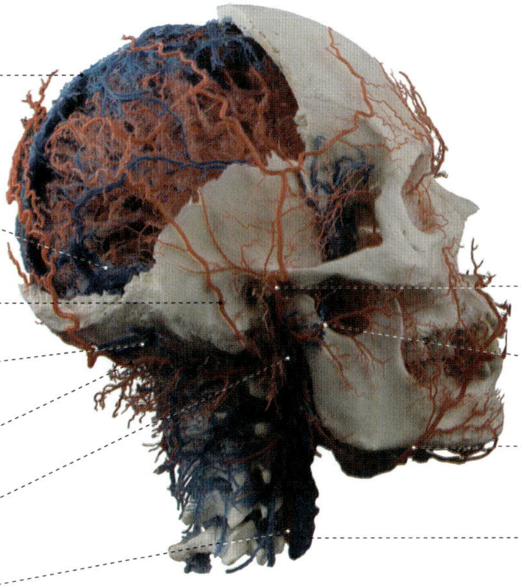

图 10–14　头部的血管铸型（外侧面观）（2）
Cast of blood vessels of head. Lateral aspect (2)

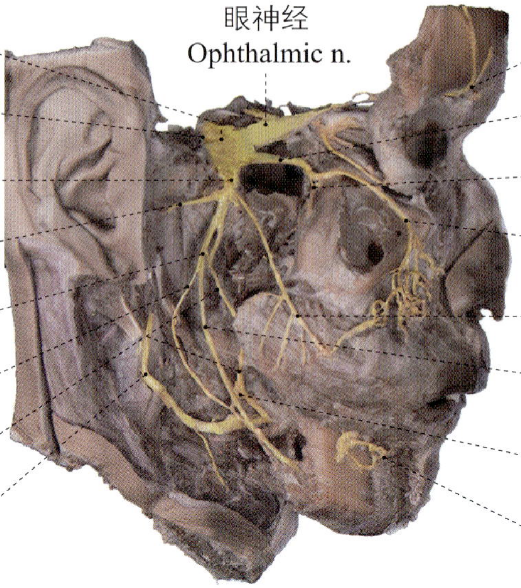

图 10–15　三叉神经（外侧面观）
Trigeminal n. Lateral aspect

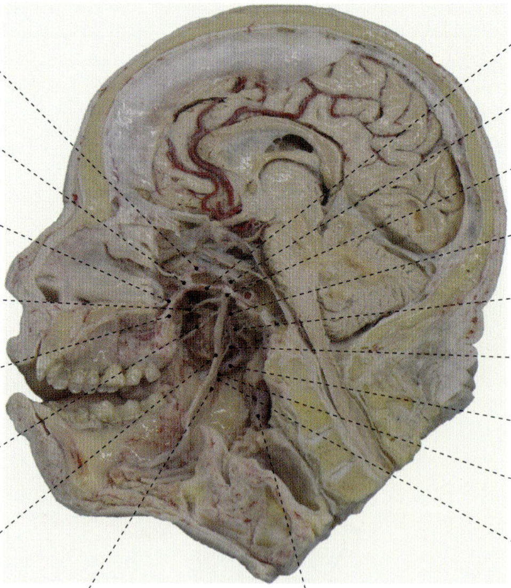

图 10–16　三叉神经（内侧面观）
Trigeminal n. Medial aspect

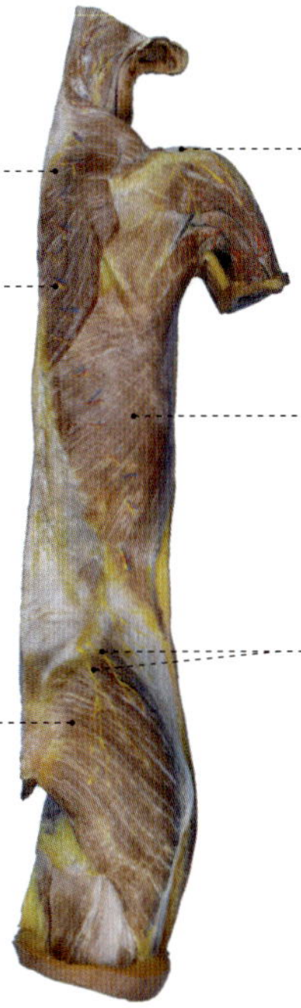

图 10–17　背部的皮神经

Cutaneous nerves of back

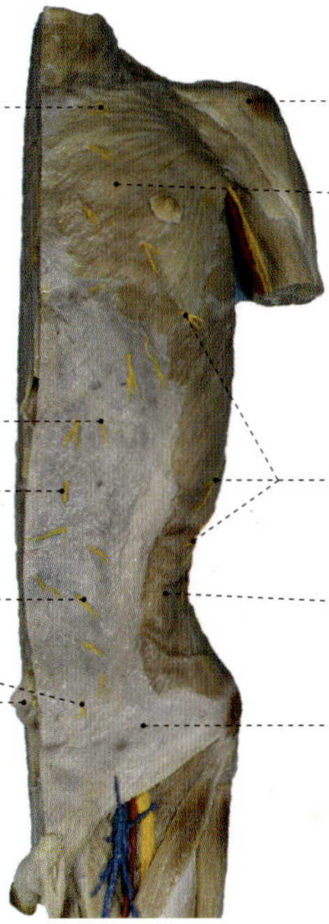

图 10–18　胸腹壁的皮神经

Cutaneous nerves of thoracic and abdominal wall

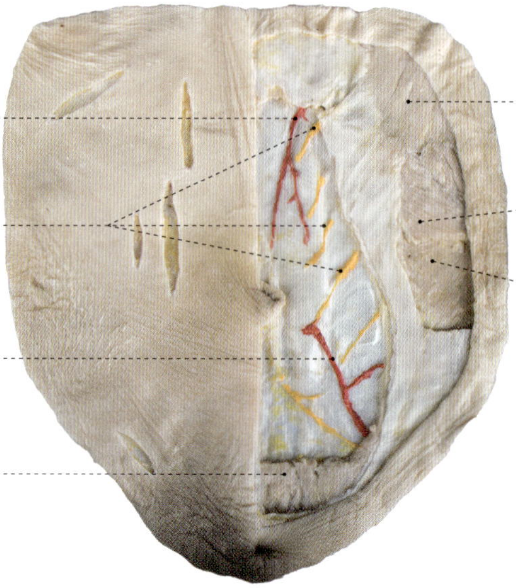

图 10-19 腹壁的肌肉、血管和神经

Muscles, blood vessels and nerves of abdominal wall

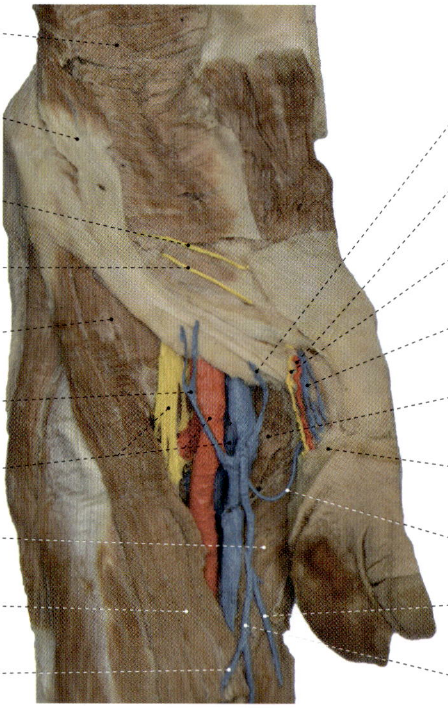

图 10-20 腹股沟区

Inguinal region

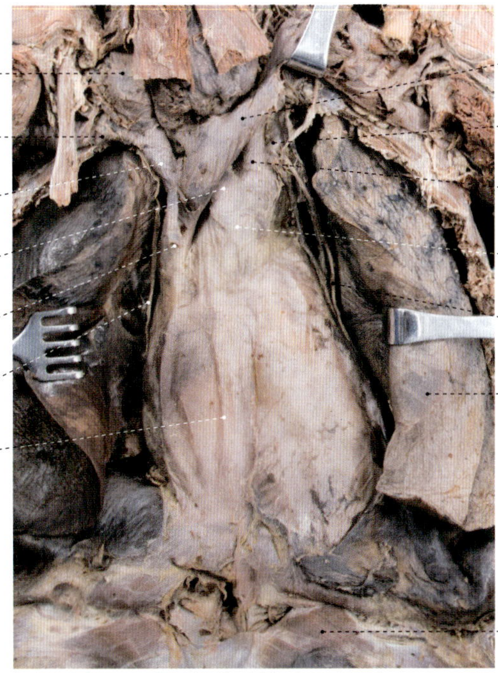

图 10–21　胸腔（前面观）（1）

The thoracic cavity. Anterior aspect (1)

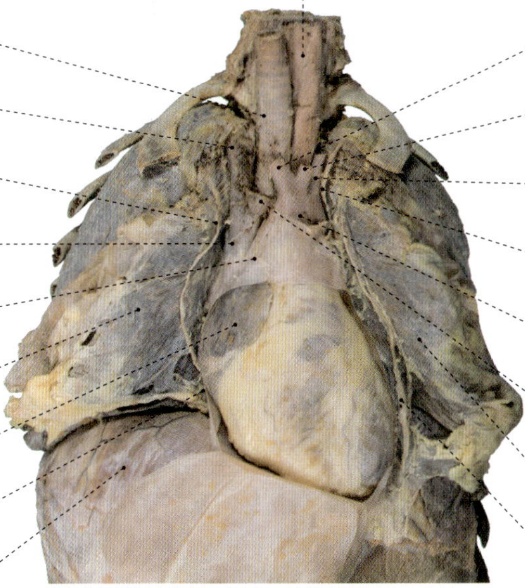

图 10–22　胸腔（前面观）（2）

The thoracic cavity. Anterior aspect (2)

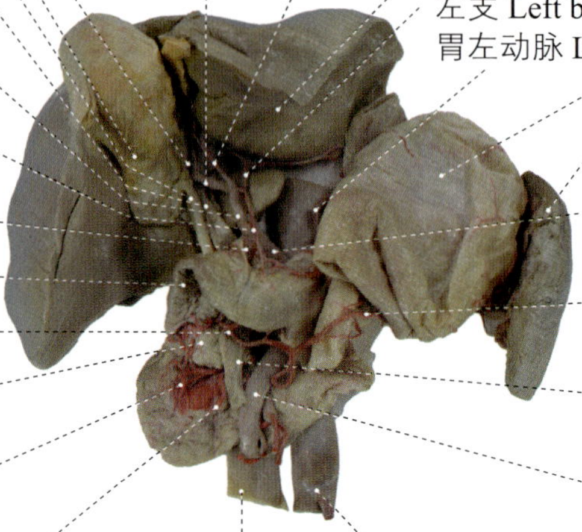

图 10–27　腹上部的器官和动脉（1）

Organs and arteries of upper abdomen (1)

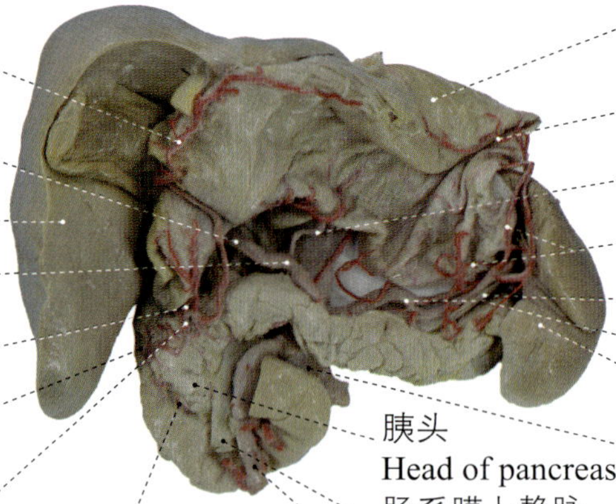

图 10–28　腹上部的器官和动脉（2）

Organs and arteries of upper abdomen (2)

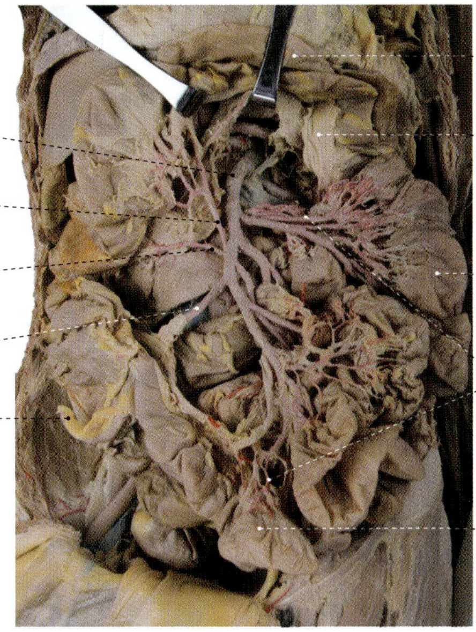

图 10–29　腹下部的器官和动脉（1）

Organs and arteries of lower abdomen (1)

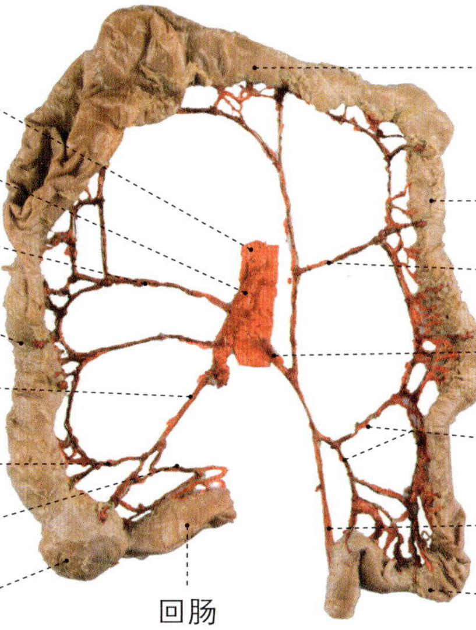

图 10–30　腹下部的器官和动脉（2）

Organs and arteries of lower abdomen (2)

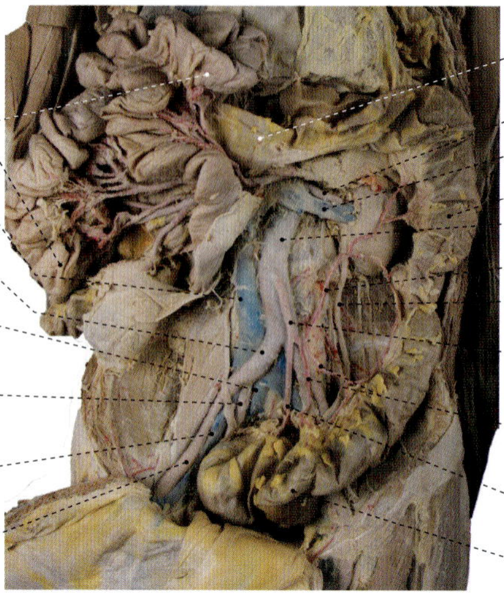

图 10–31　腹下部的器官和血管（3）
Organs and blood vessels of lower abdomen (3)

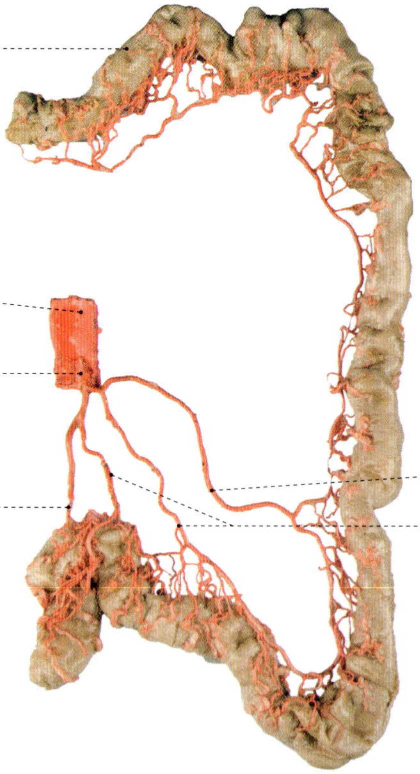

图 10–32　腹下部的器官和动脉（4）
Organs and arteries of lower abdomen (4)

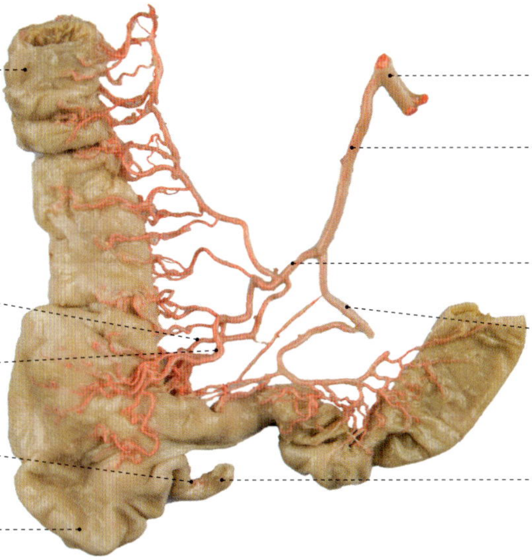

图 10–33　回盲部的动脉

Arteries of ileocecal region

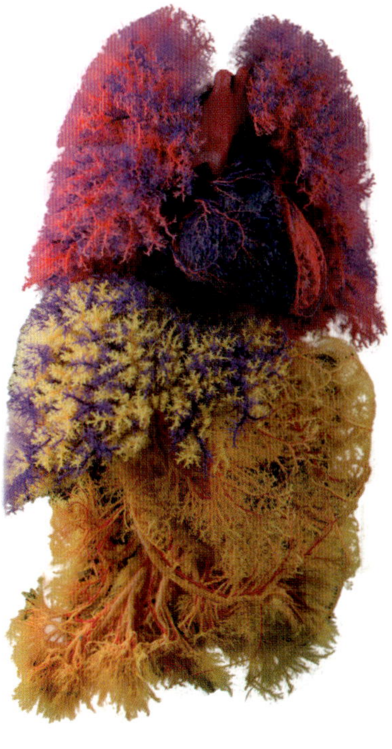

心—蓝色：右心房和右心室

红色：左心房和左心室

红色：冠状动脉

Heart—blue: right atrium and ventricle red: left atrium and ventricle red: left and right coronary a.

肺—蓝色：肺动脉

红色：肺静脉

Lung—blue：pulmonary a. red: pulmonary v.

肝—红色：肝固有动脉

黄色：肝门静脉及其分支

蓝色：肝静脉

Liver—red: proper hepatic a.   yellow: hepatic portal v. and its branches

胃—红色：动脉

黄色：肝门静脉属支

Stomach—red: arteries: tributaries of hepatic portal v.

图 10–34　心、肺、肝和胃的铸型（前面观）

Cast of heart, lungs, liver and stomach. Anterior aspect

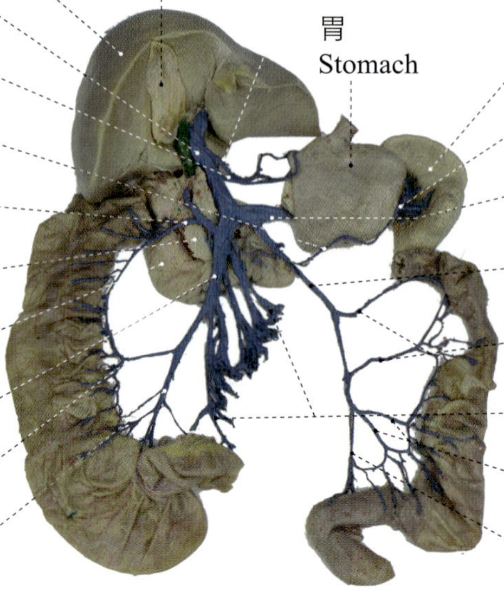

图 10–35　肝门静脉及其属支

Hepatic portal v. and its tributaries

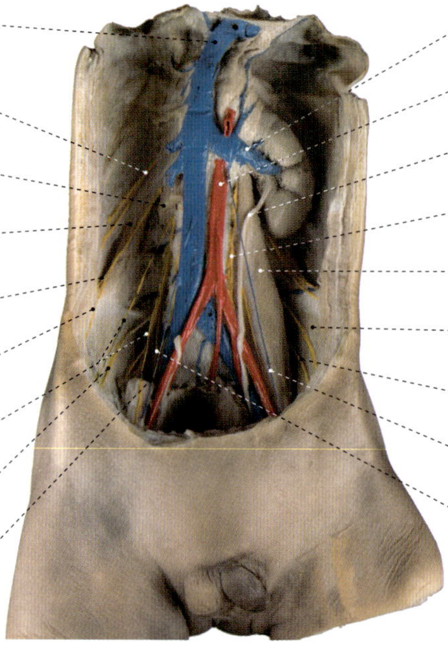

图 10–36　腹后壁的血管和神经（前面观）

Blood vessels and nerves of posterior abdominal wall. Anterior aspect

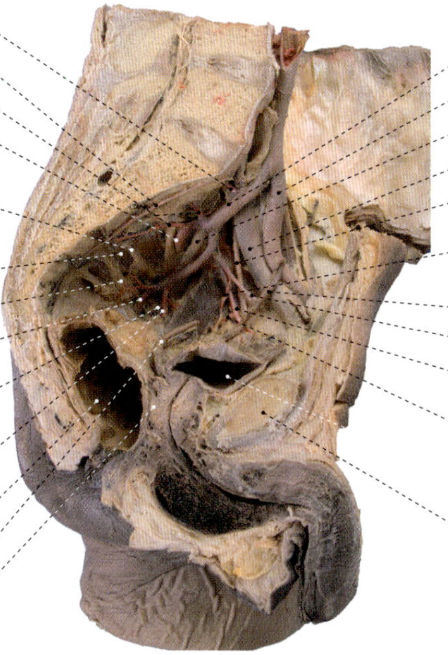

图 10–37　盆腔的血管和神经（男性）

Blood vessels and nerves of pelvic cavity (male)

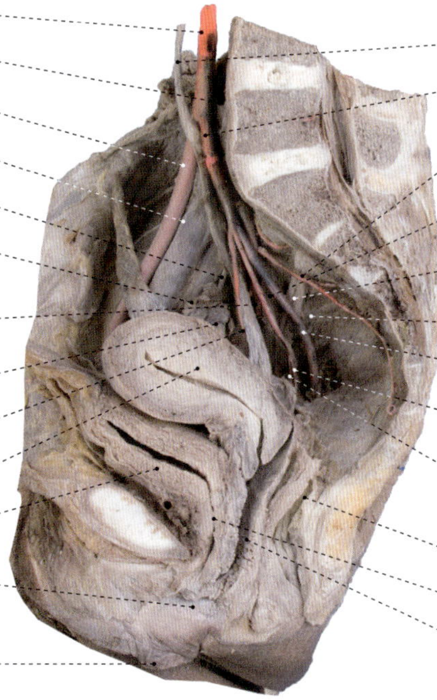

图 10–38　盆腔的血管和神经（女性）

Blood vessels and nerves of pelvic cavity (female)

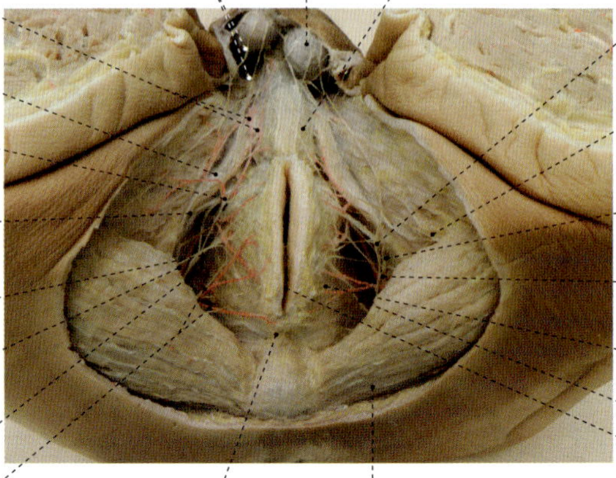

图 10–39　男性会阴的肌肉、血管及神经

Muscles, blood vessels and nerves of male perineum

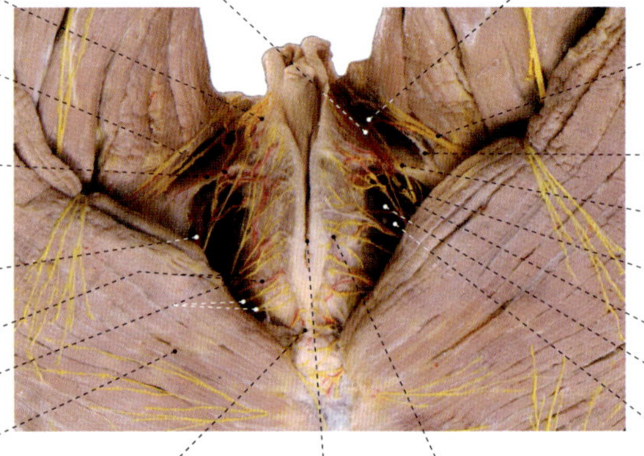

图 10–40　女性会阴的肌肉、血管及神经

Muscles, blood vessels and nerves of female perineum

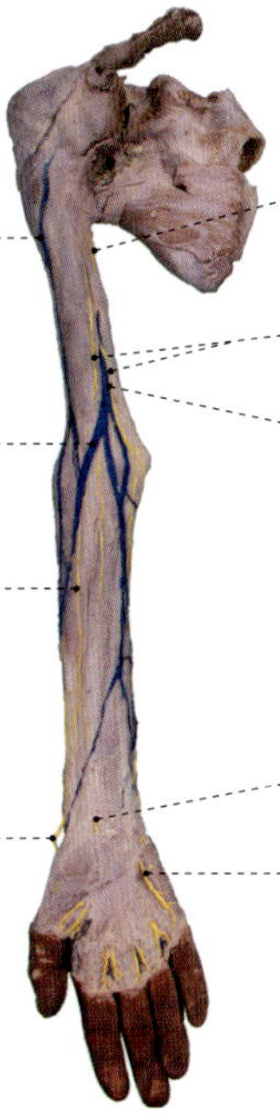

图 10–41 上肢的浅静脉和皮神经（前面观）

Superficial veins and cutaneous nerves of upper limb. Anterior aspect

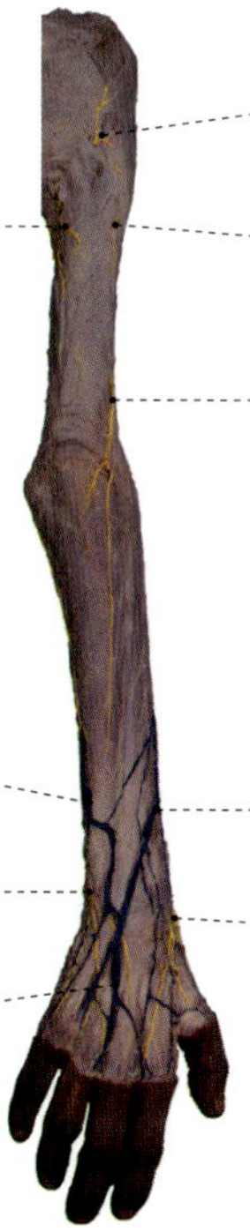

图 10–42 上肢的浅静脉和皮神经（后面观）

Superficial veins and cutaneous nerves of upper limb. Posterior aspect

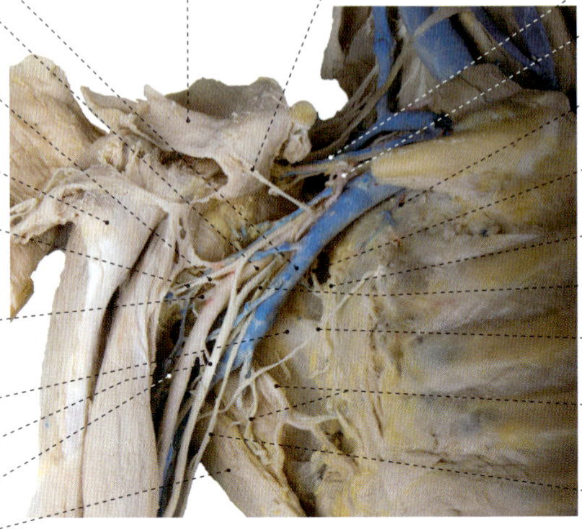

图 10–43 腋窝的血管和神经（1）

Blood vessels and nerves of axillary fossa (1)

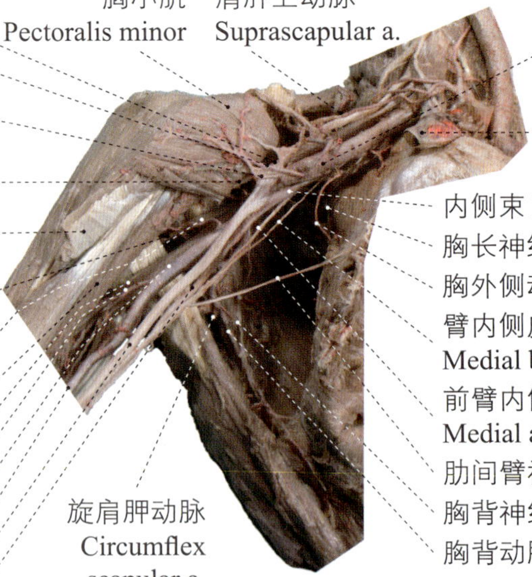

图 10–44 腋窝的血管和神经（2）

Blood vessels and nerves of axillary fossa (2)

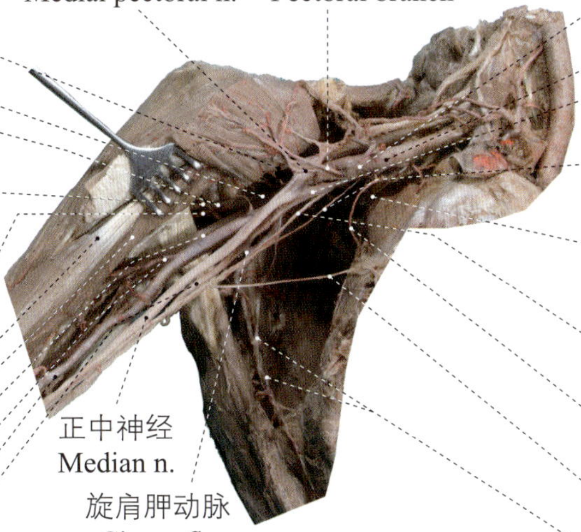

图 10–45　腋窝的血管和神经（3）

Blood vessels and nerves of axillary fossa (3)

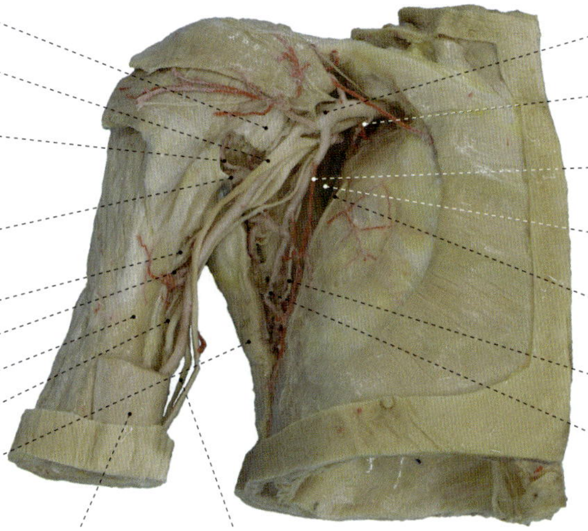

图 10–46　腋窝的血管和神经（4）

Blood vessels and nerves of axillary fossa (4)

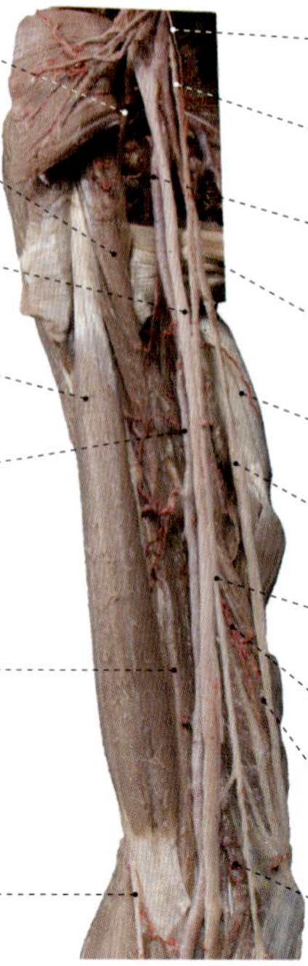

图 10–47　臂部的肌肉、血管和神经（前面观）（1）

Muscles, blood vessels and nerves of arm. Anterior aspect (1)

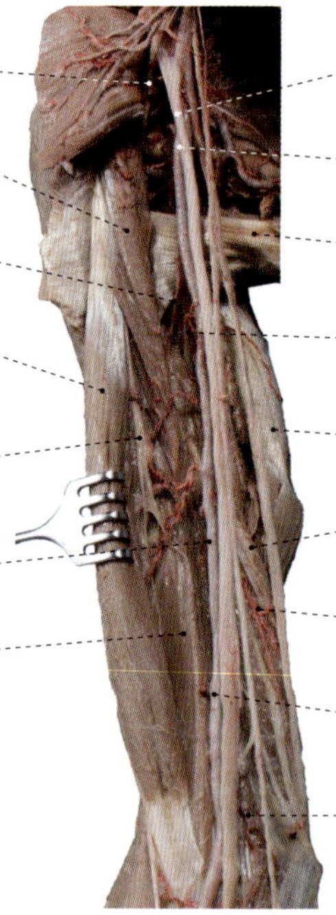

图 10–48　臂部的肌肉、血管和神经（前面观）（2）

Muscles, blood vessels and nerves of arm. Anterior aspect (2)

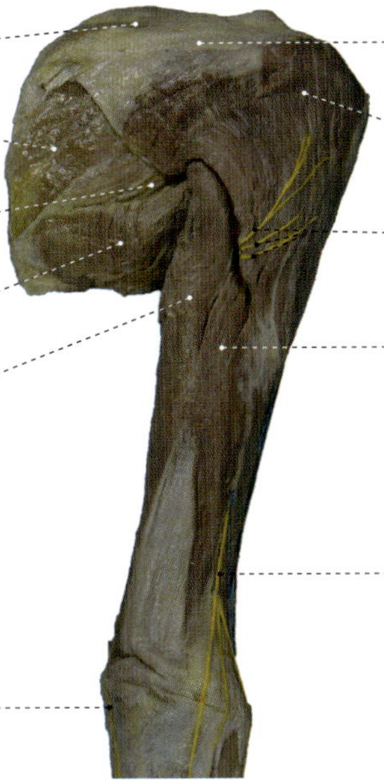

图 10–49　肩、臂部的肌肉、血管和神经（后面观）（1）

Muscles, blood vessels and nerves of shoulder and arm. Posterior aspect (1)

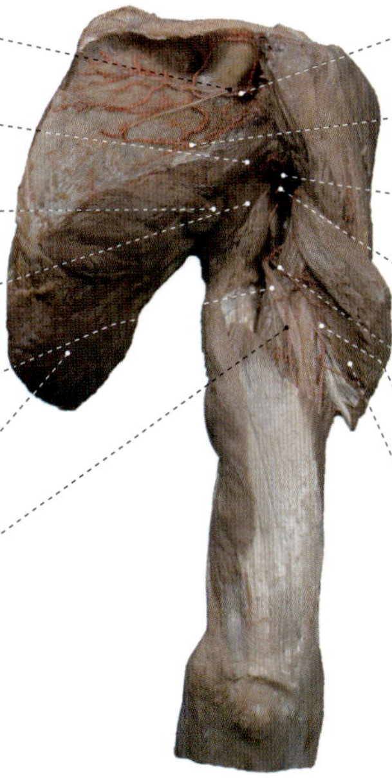

图 10–50　肩、臂部的肌肉、血管和神经（后面观）（2）

Muscles, blood vessels and nerves of shoulder and arm. Posterior aspect (2)

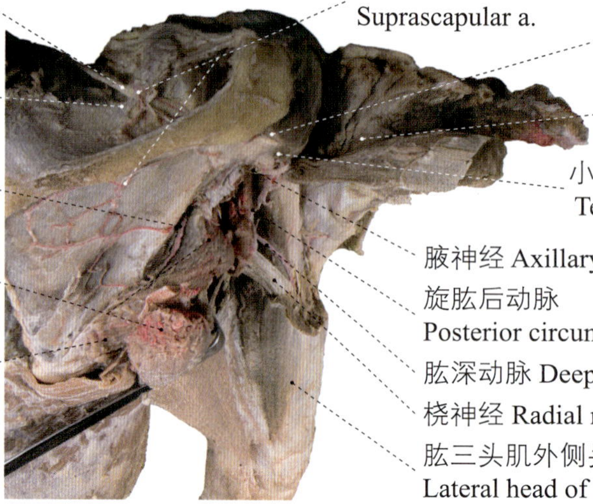

图 10–51　肩、臂部的肌肉、血管和神经（后面观）（3）

Muscles, blood vessels and nerves of shoulder and arm. Posterior aspect (3)

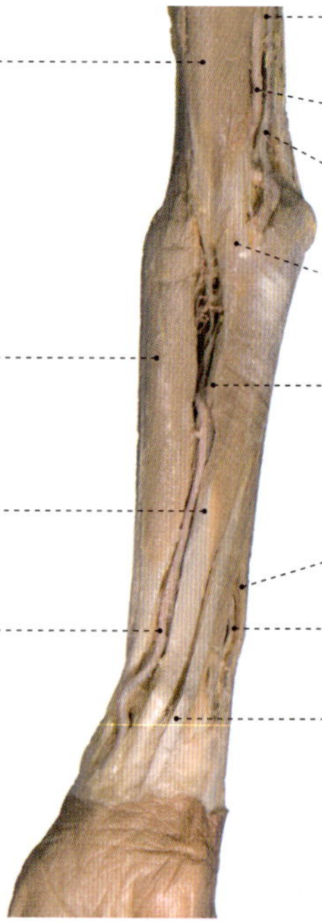

图 10–52　前臂的肌肉、血管和神经（前面观）（1）

Muscles, blood vessels and nerves of forearm. Anterior aspect (1)

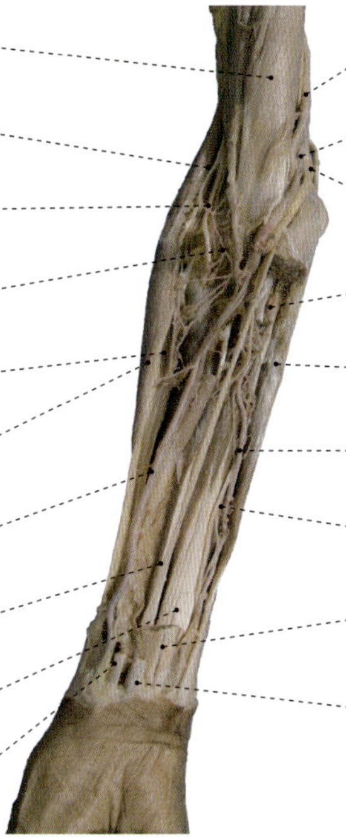

图 10–53　前臂的肌肉、血管和神经（前面观）（2）

Muscles, blood vessels and nerves of forearm. Anterior aspect (2)

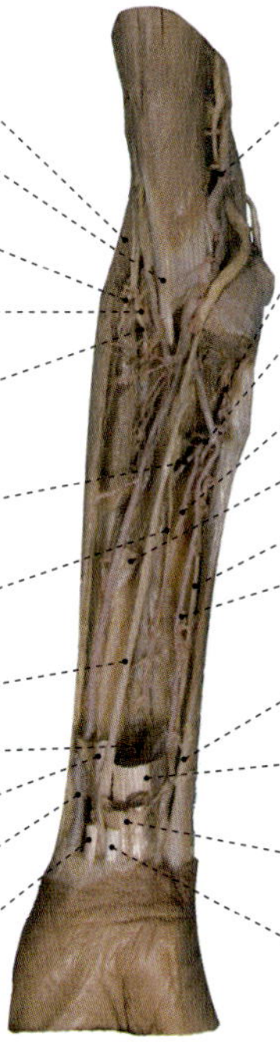

图 10–54　前臂的肌肉、血管和神经（前面观）（3）

Muscles, blood vessels and nerves of forearm. Anterior aspect (3)

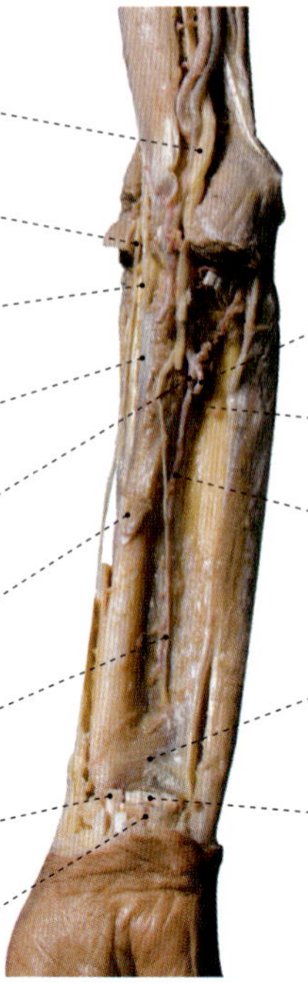

图 10-55　前臂的肌肉、血管和神经（前面观）（4）

Muscles, blood vessels and nerves of forearm. Anterior aspect (4)

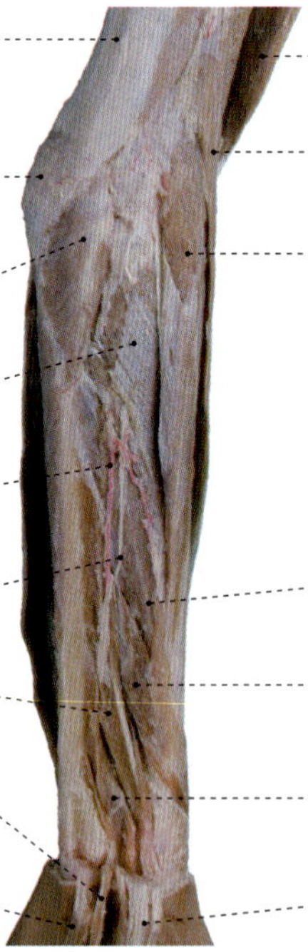

图 10-56　前臂的肌肉、血管和神经（后面观）

Muscles, blood vessels and nerves of the forearm. Posterior aspect

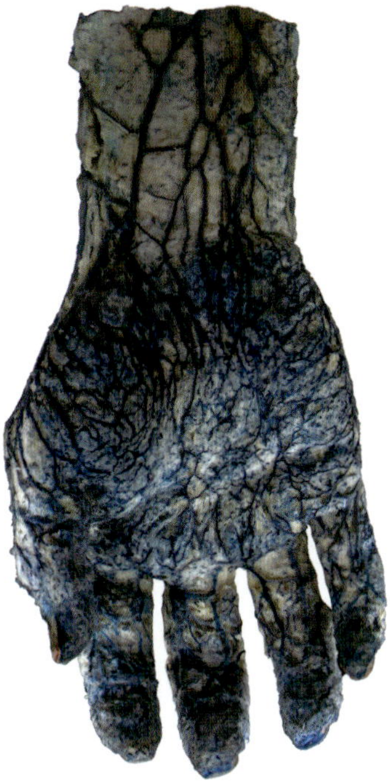

图 10–57　手掌的浅静脉
Superficial veins of palm of hand

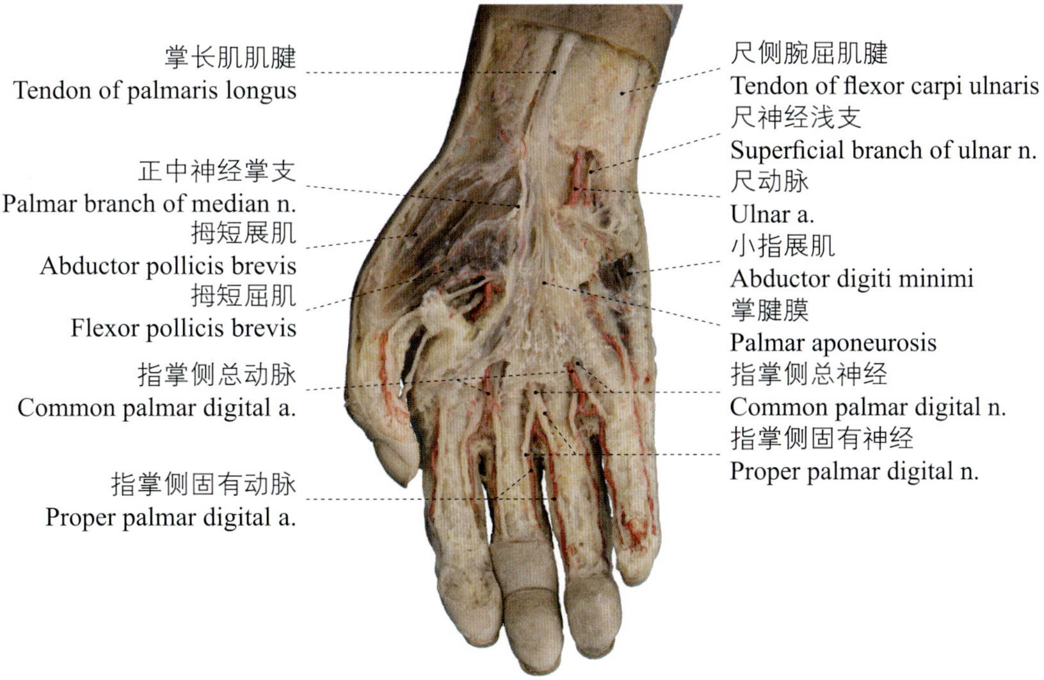

图 10–58　手的肌肉、血管和神经（掌侧面观）（1）
Muscles, blood vessels and nerves of hand. Palmar aspect (1)

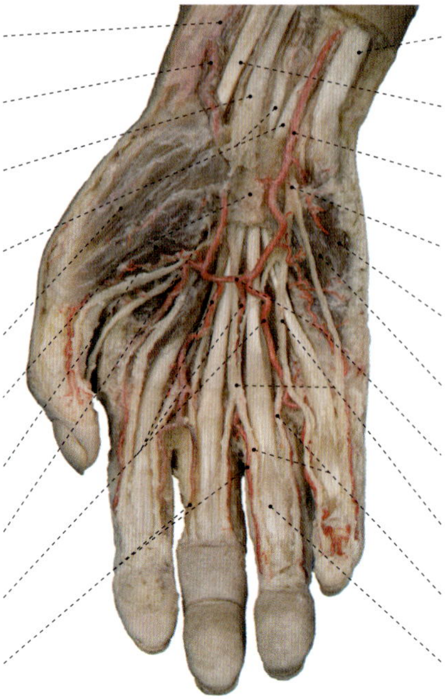

图 10–59　手的肌肉、血管和神经（掌侧面观）（2）

Muscles, blood vessels and nerves of hand. Palmar aspect (2)

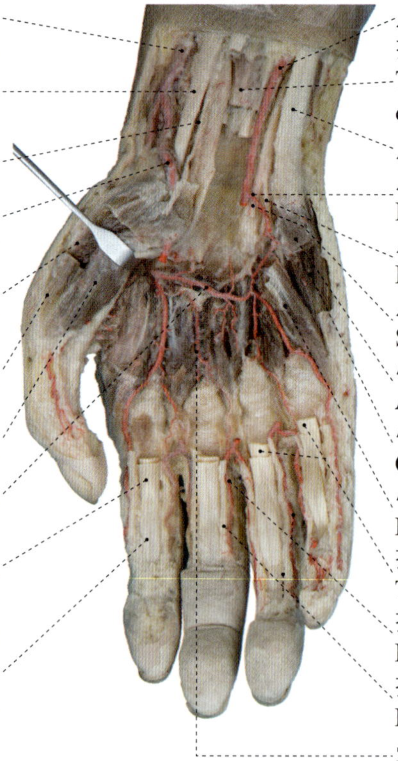

图 10–60　手的肌肉、血管和神经（掌侧面观）（3）

Muscles, blood vessels and nerves of hand. Palmar aspect (3)

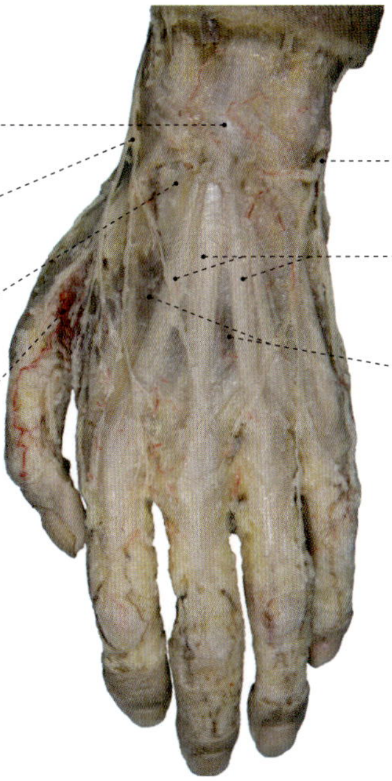

图 10-61　手的血管、神经（背面观）（1）
Blood vessels and nerves of hand. Dorsal aspect (1)

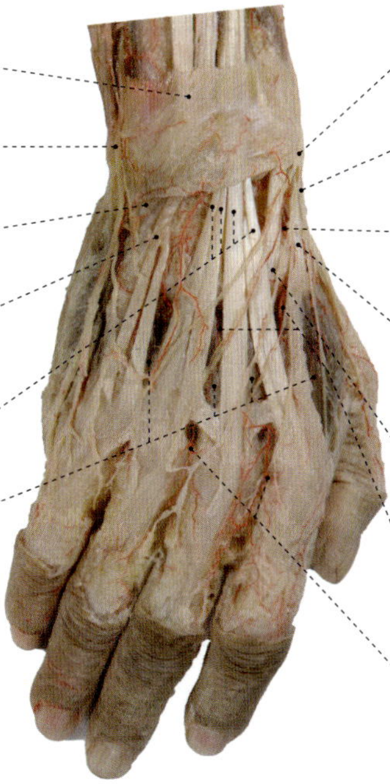

图 10-62　手的血管、神经（背面观）（2）
Blood vessels and nerves of hand. Dorsal aspect (2)

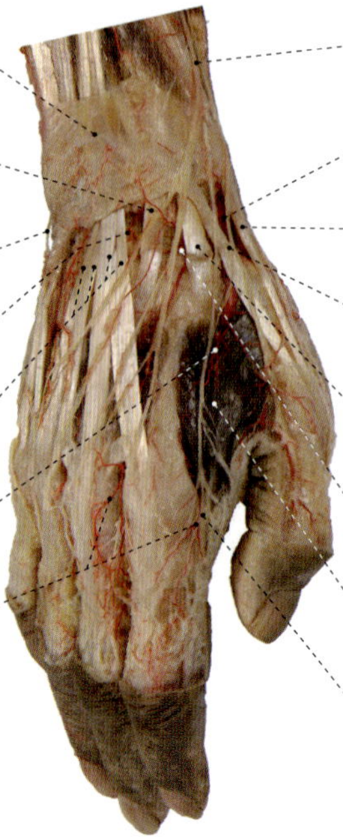

图 10–63　手的血管、神经（背外侧面观）

Blood vessels and nerves of hand. Dorsal and lateral aspect

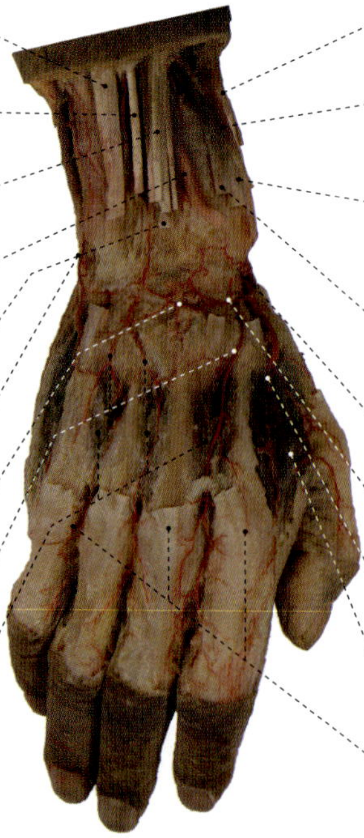

图 10–64　手的血管、神经（背面观）（3）

Blood vessels and nerves of hand. Dorsal aspect (3)

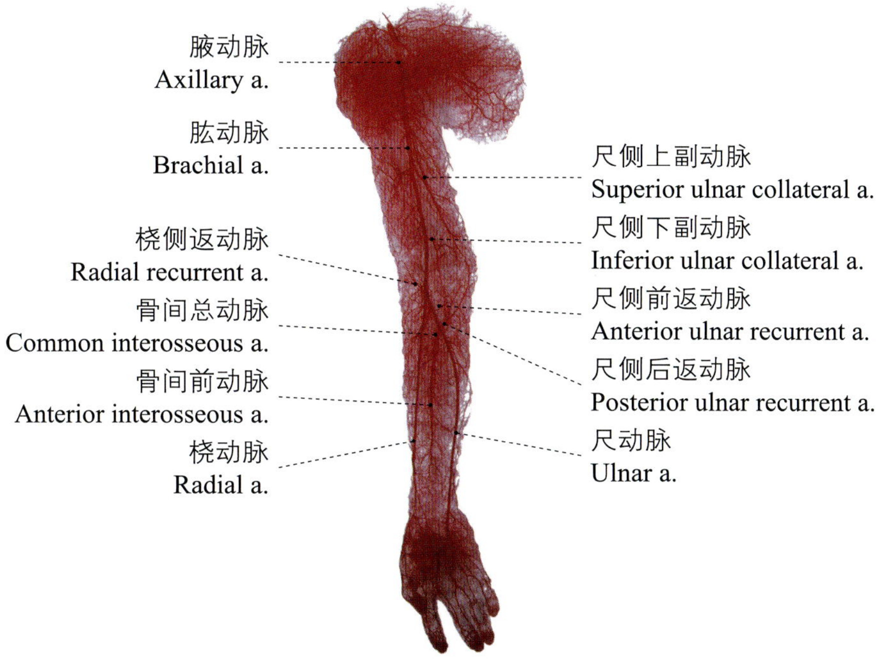

图 10-65　上肢的动脉铸型（前面观）
Cast of arteries of upper limb. Anterior aspect

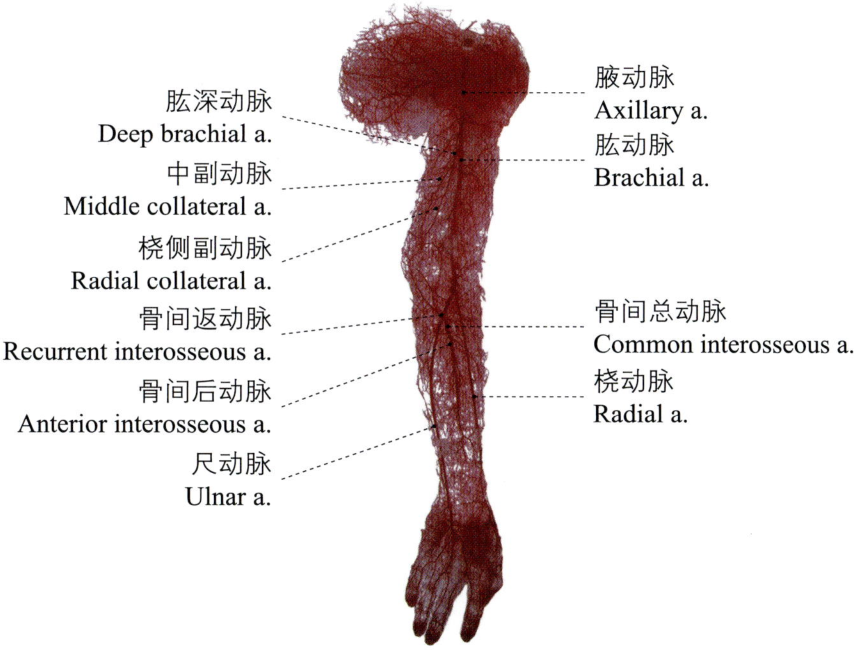

图 10-66　上肢的动脉铸型（后面观）
Cast of arteries of upper limb. Posterior aspect

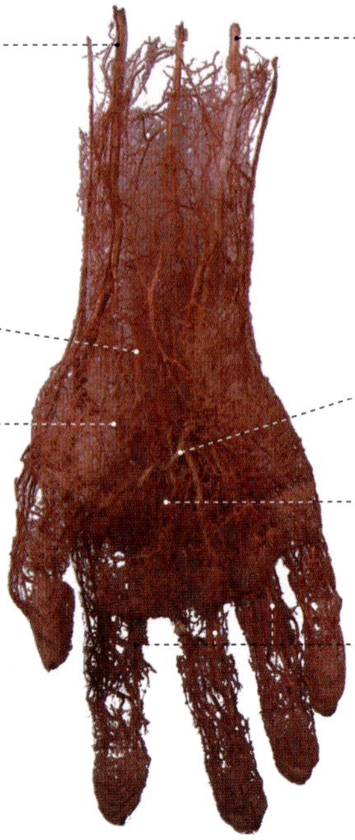

图 10-67　手的动脉铸型（前面观）
Cast of arteries of hand. Anterior aspect

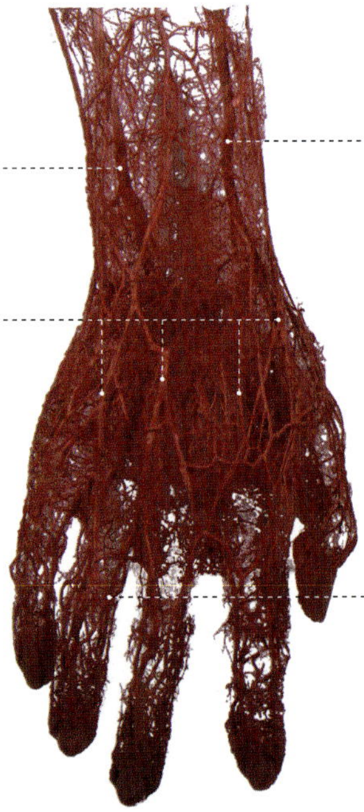

图 10-68　手的动脉铸型（后面观）
Cast of arteries of hand. Posterior aspect

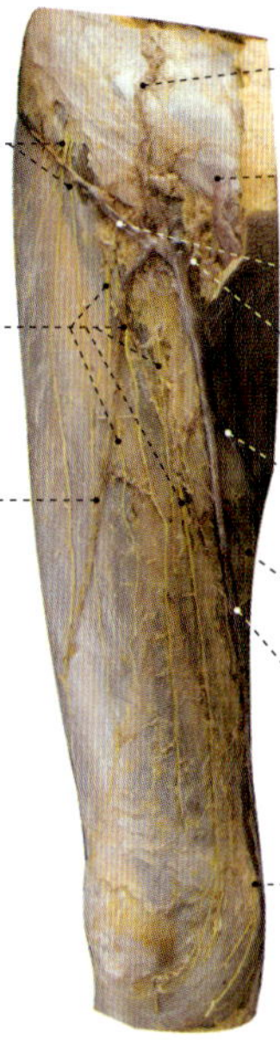

图 10–69　大腿的浅静脉和皮神经（前面观）
Superficial veins and cutaneous nerves of thigh. Anterior aspect

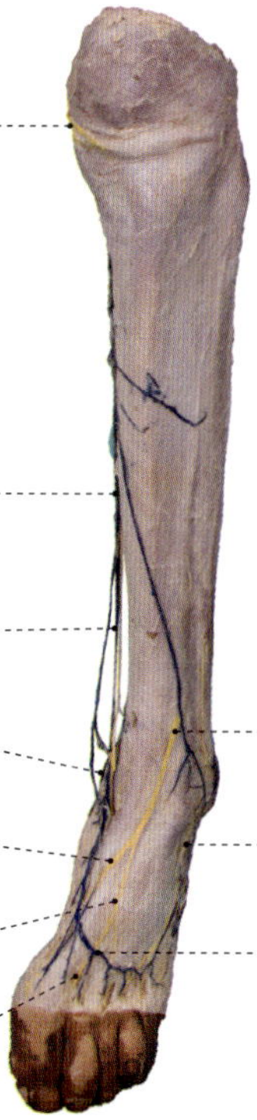

图 10–70　小腿的浅静脉和皮神经（前面观）
Superficial veins and cutaneous nerves of leg. Anterior aspect

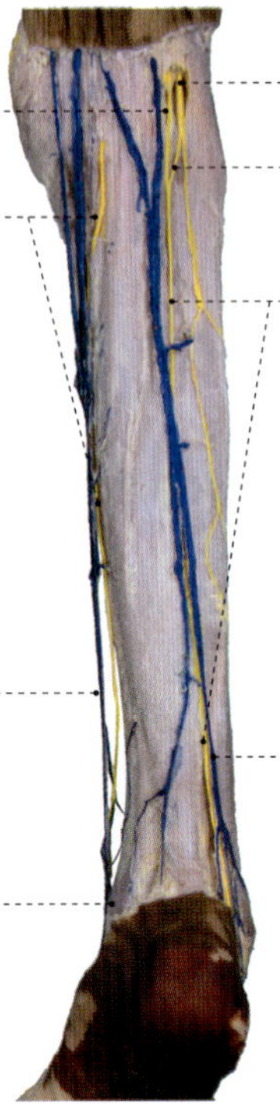

图 10–71 小腿的浅静脉和皮神经（后面观）
Superficial veins and cutaneous nerves of leg. Posterior aspect

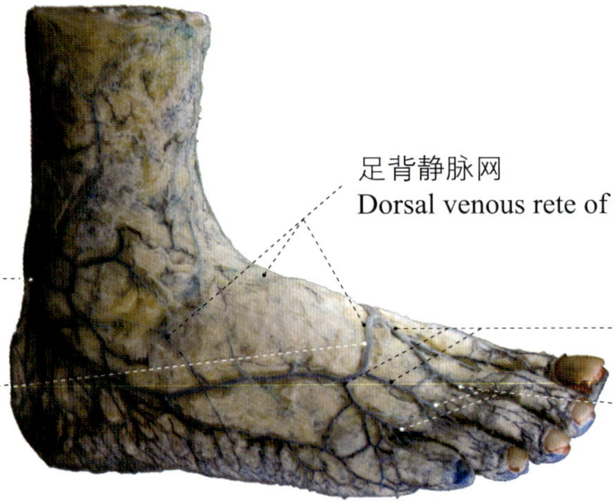

图 10–72 足背的浅静脉（外侧面观）
Superficial veins of dorsum of foot. Lateral aspect

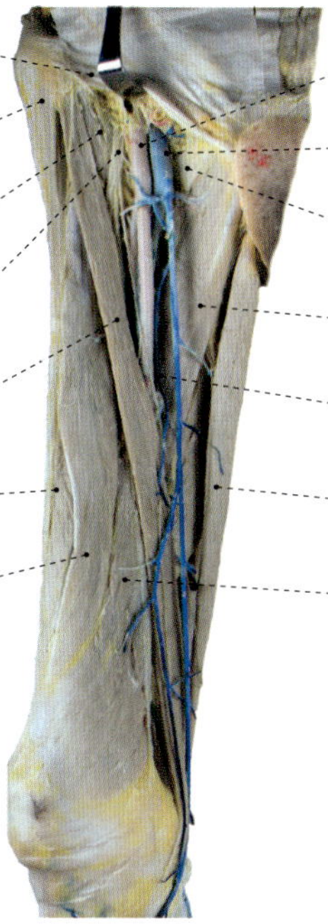

图 10–73　股前区的肌肉、血管和神经（1）

Muscles, blood vessels and nerves of anterior region of thigh (1)

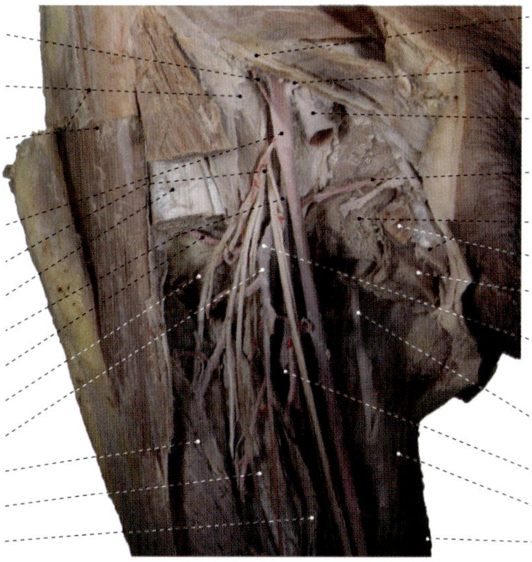

图 10–74　股前区的肌肉、血管和神经（2）

Muscles, blood vessels and nerves of anterior region of thigh (2)

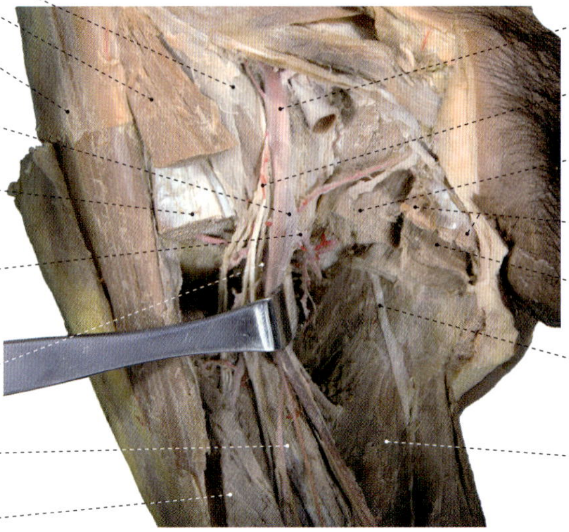

图 10–75　股前区的肌肉、血管和神经（3）

Muscles，blood vessels and nerves of anterior region of the thigh (3)

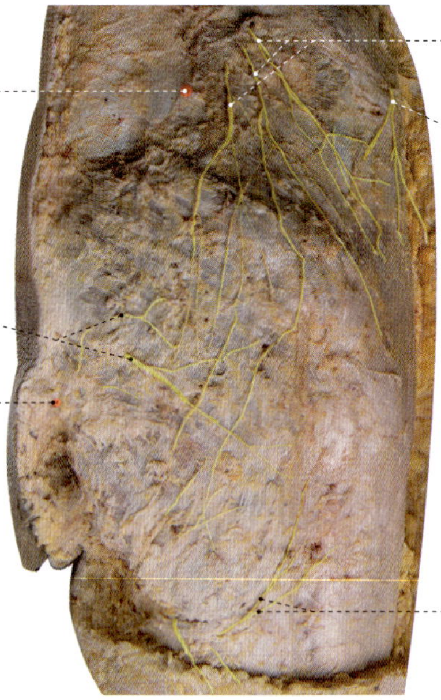

图 10–76　臀区的皮神经

Cutaneous n. of gluteal region

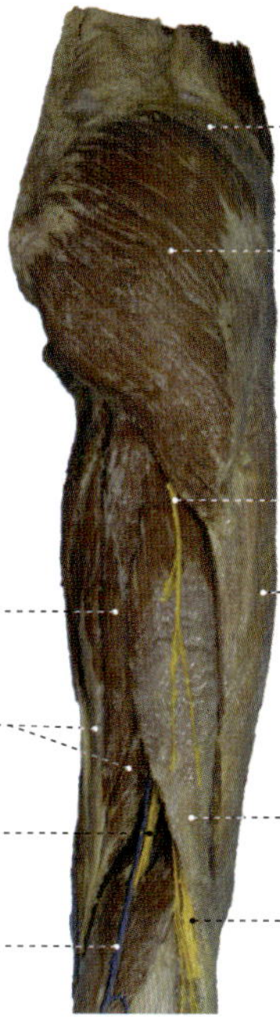

图 10–77　臀区和股后区的肌肉、血管和神经（1）

Muscles, blood vessels and nerves of gluteal region and posterior region of thigh (1)

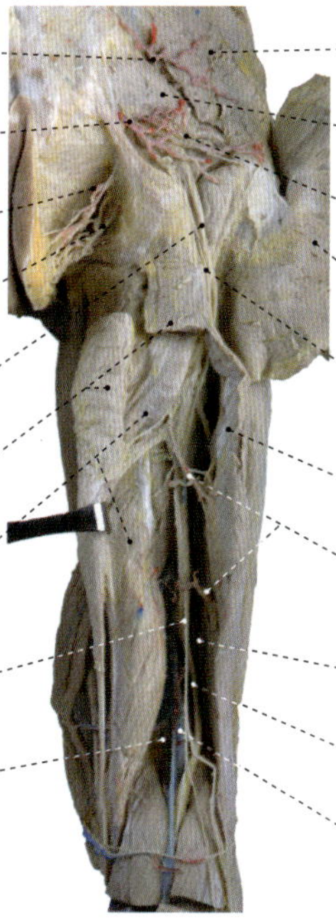

图 10–78　臀区和股后区的肌肉、血管和神经（2）

Muscles, blood vessels and nerves of gluteal region and posterior region of thigh (2)

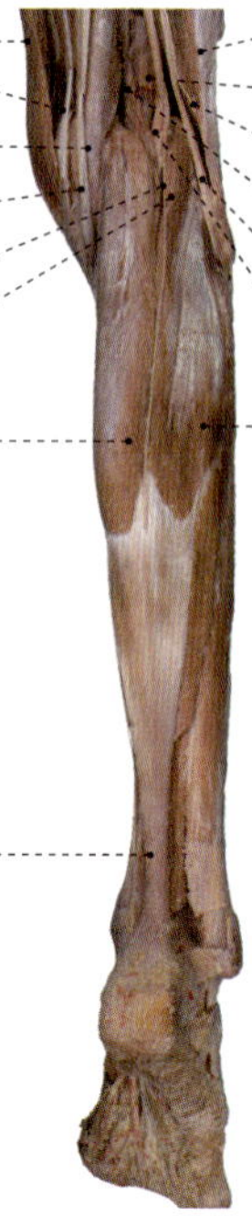

图 10–83　小腿的肌肉、血管和神经（后面观）（1）

Muscles, blood vessels and nerves of leg. Posterior aspect (1)

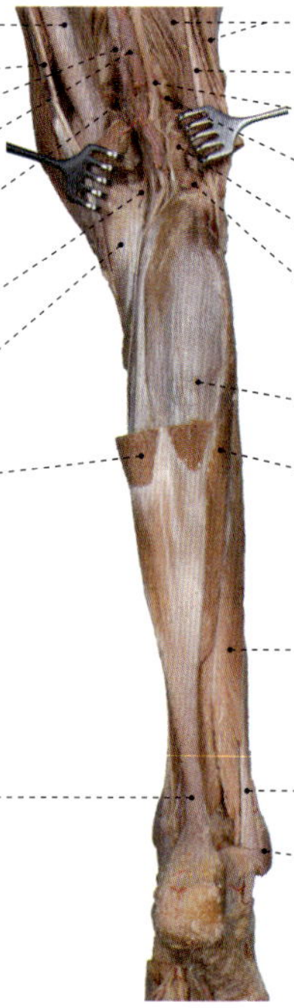

图 10–84　小腿的肌肉、血管和神经（后面观）（2）

Muscles, blood vessels and nerves of leg. Posterior aspect (2)

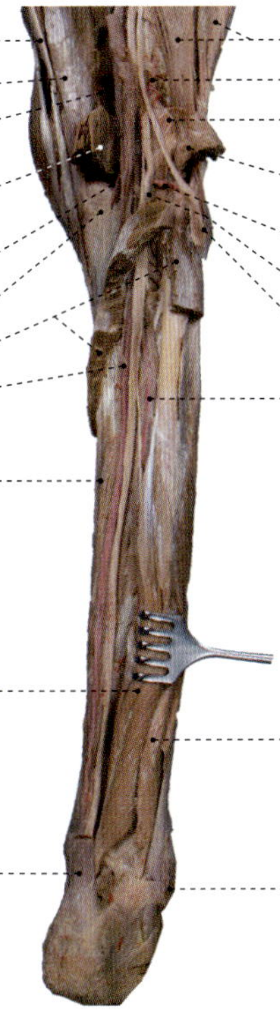

图 10–85　小腿的肌肉、血管和神经（后面观）（3）
Muscles, blood vessels and nerves of leg. Posterior aspect (3)

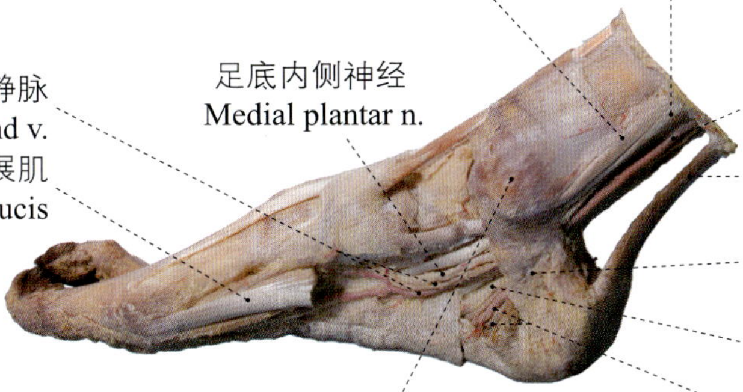

图 10–86　足的内侧面观
Medial aspect of foot

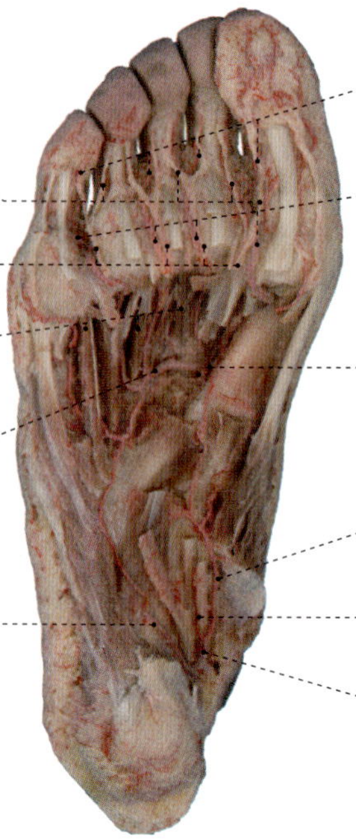

图 10–91　足底的肌肉、血管

Muscles, blood vessels of sole of foot

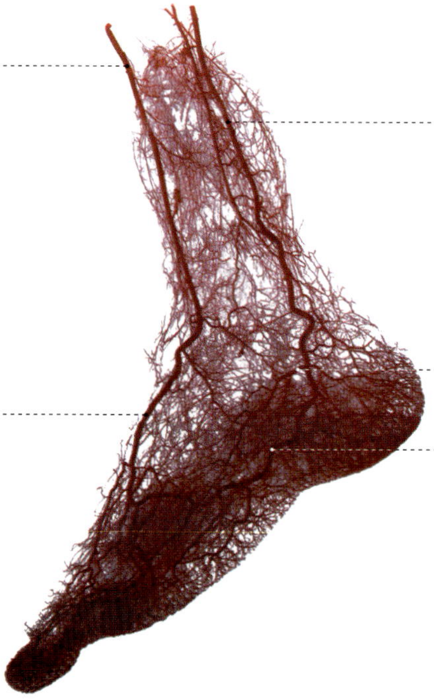

图 10–92　足的动脉铸型

Cast of arteries of foot

第十一章　头部、躯干和四肢断面

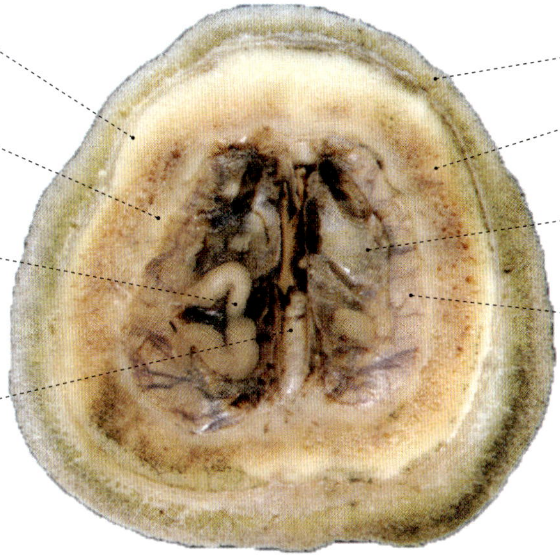

图 11-1　经上矢状窦的横断面

Transverse section through superior sagittal sinus

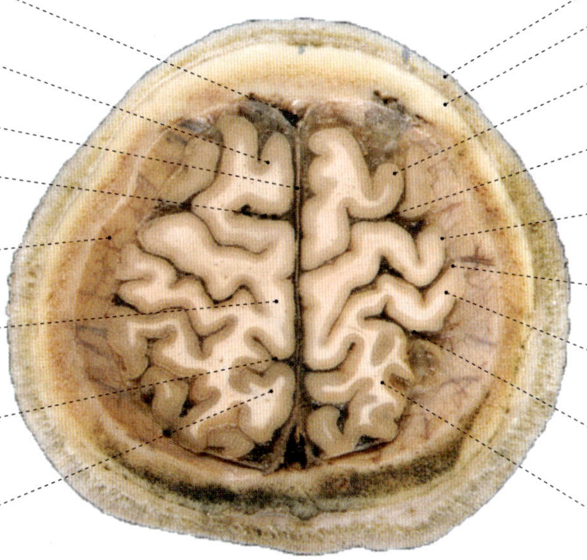

图 11-2　经中央旁小叶上份的横断面

Transverse section through upper part of paracentral lobule

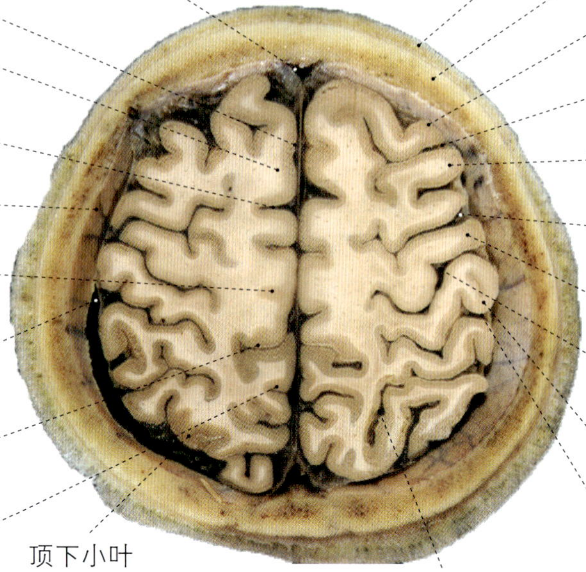

图 11–3　经中央旁小叶下份的横断面

Transverse section through lower part of paracentral lobule

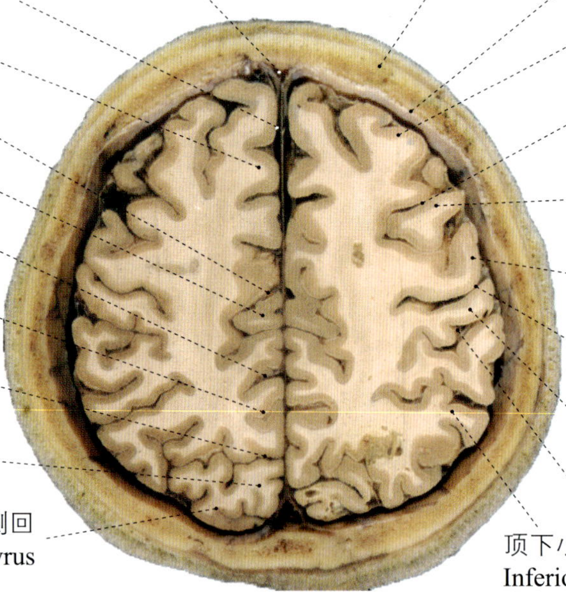

图 11–4　经顶枕沟上份的横断面

Transverse section through upper part of parietooccipital sulcus

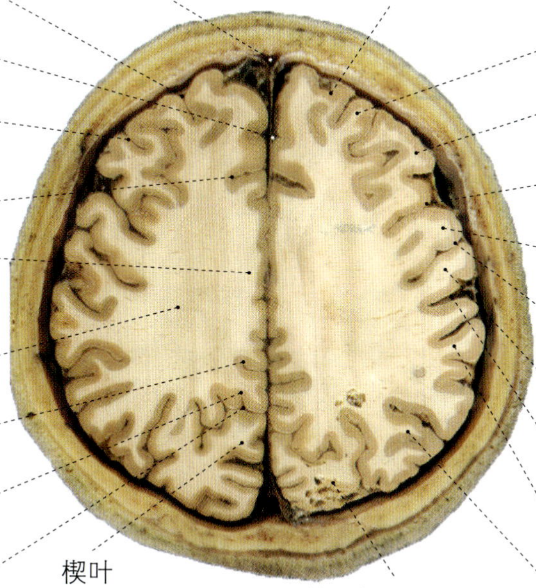

图 11–5　经半卵圆中心的横断面

Transverse section through centrum semiovale

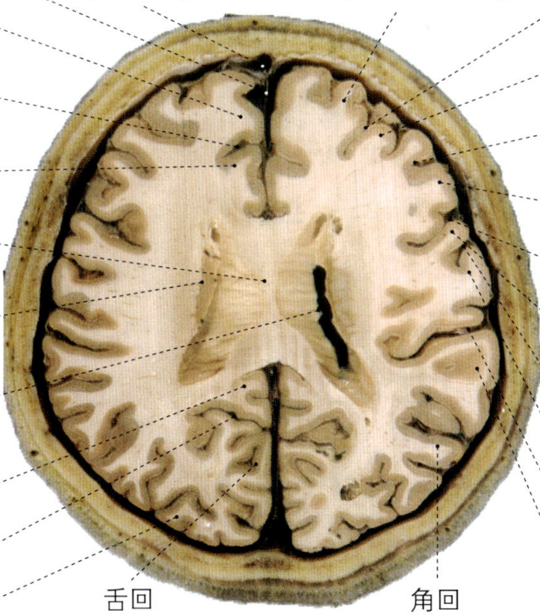

图 11–6　经胼胝体干的横断面

Transverse section through trunk of corpus callosum

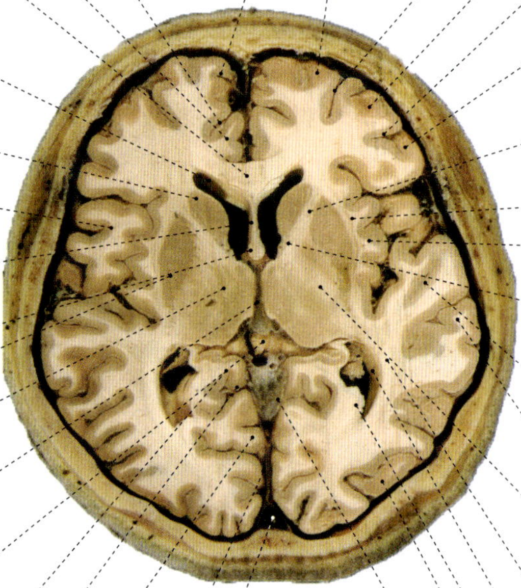

图 11–7　经胼胝体压部的横断面

Transverse section through splenium of corpus callosum

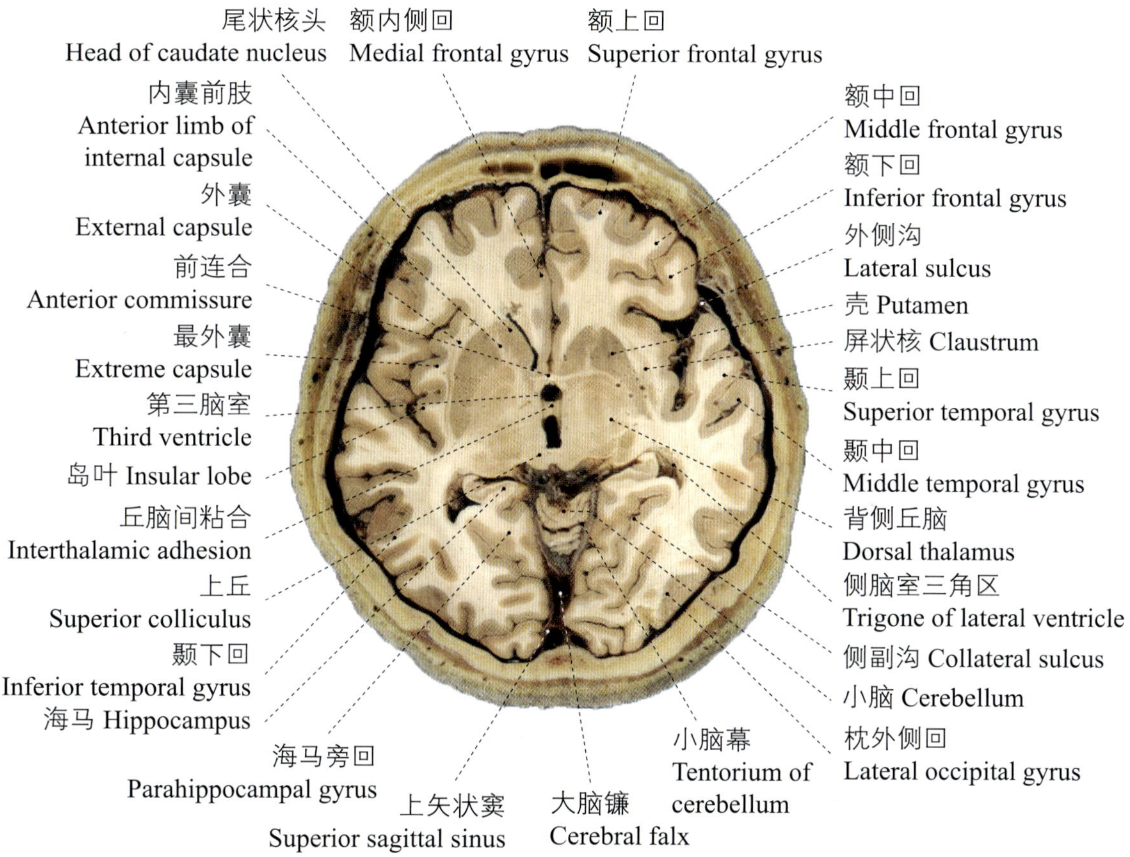

图 11-8　经前连合的横断面

Transverse section through anterior commissure

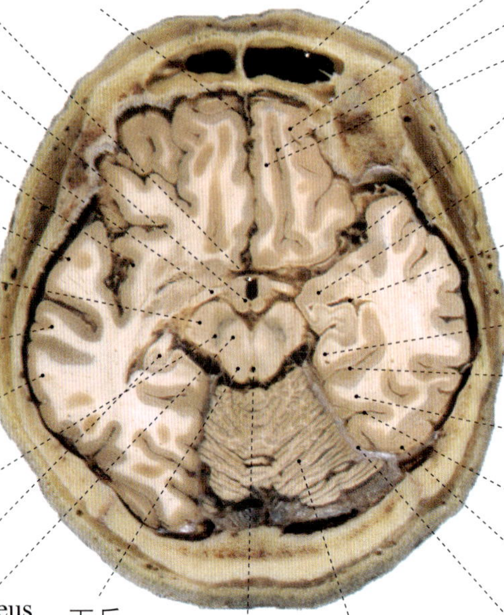

图 11–9　经红核和黑质的横断面

Transverse section through red nucleus and substantia nigra

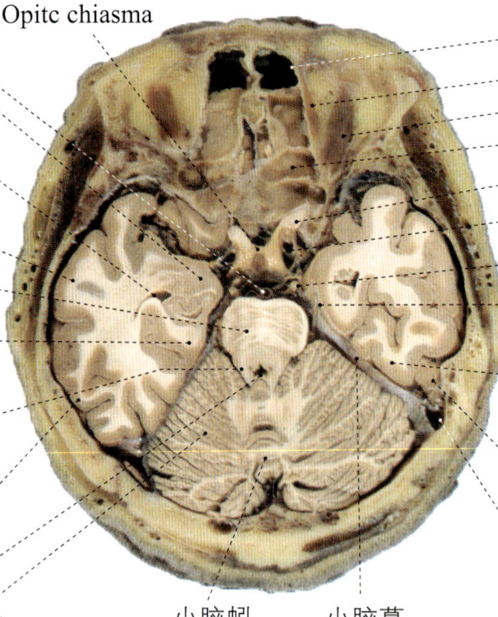

图 11–10　经小脑上脚的横断面

Transverse section through superior cerebellar peduncle

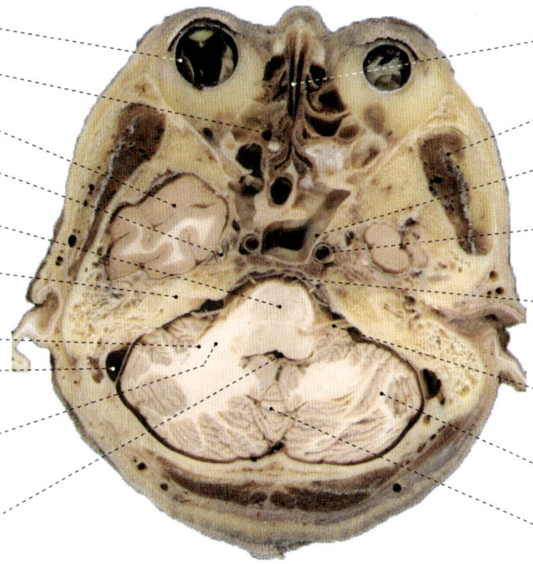

图 11–11　经小脑中脚的横断面

Transverse section through middle cerebellar peduncle

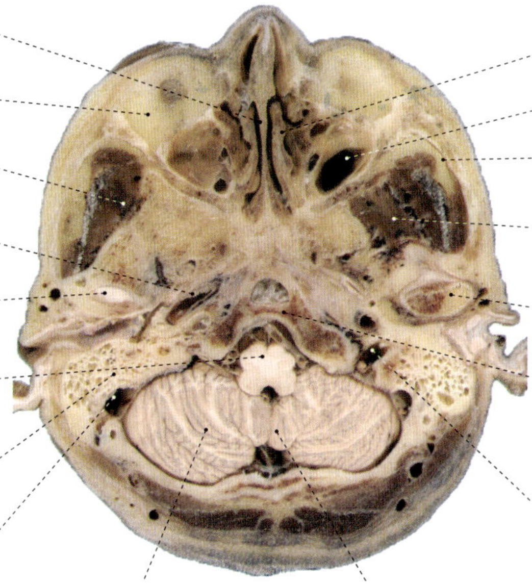

图 11–12　经颈动脉管的横断面

Transverse section through carotid canal

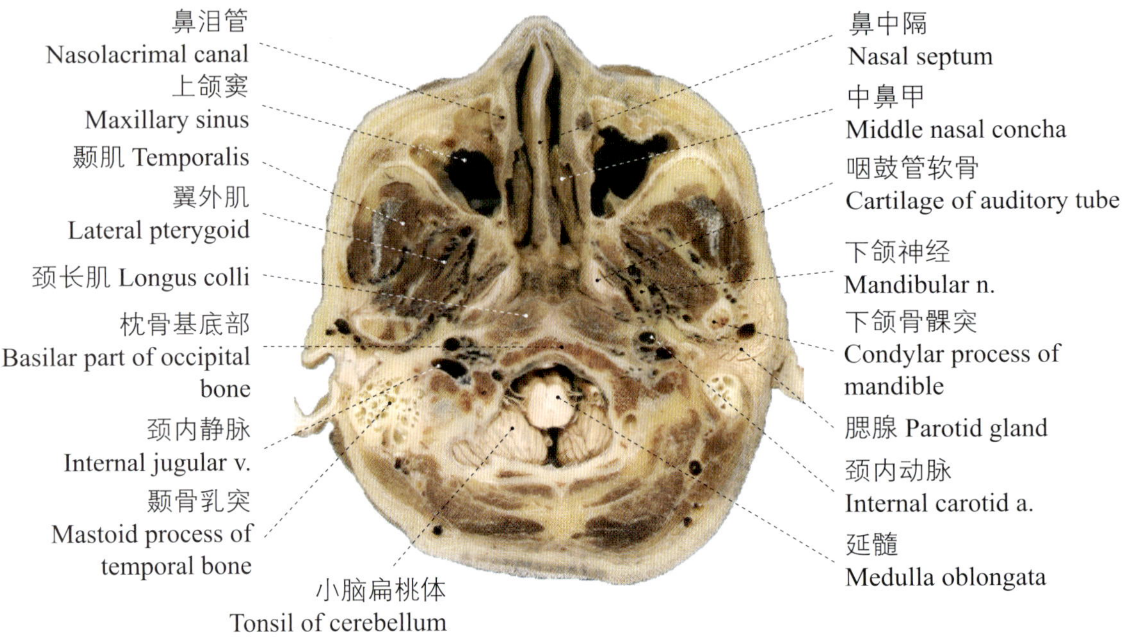

图 11-13　经小脑扁桃体的横断面

Transverse section through tonsil of cerebellum

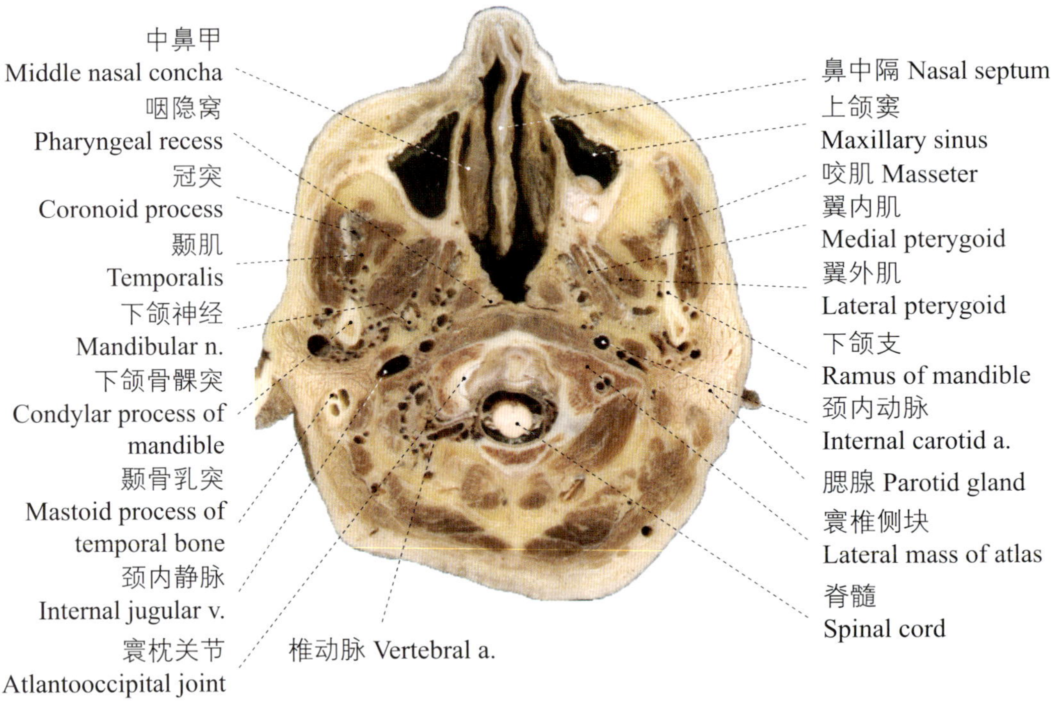

图 11-14　经寰枕关节的横断面

Transverse section through atlantooccipital joint

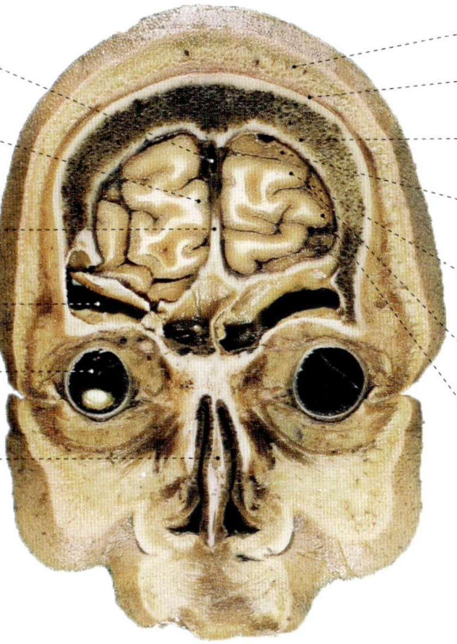

图 11-15　经额窦前份的冠状断面

Coronal section through anterior part of frontal sinus

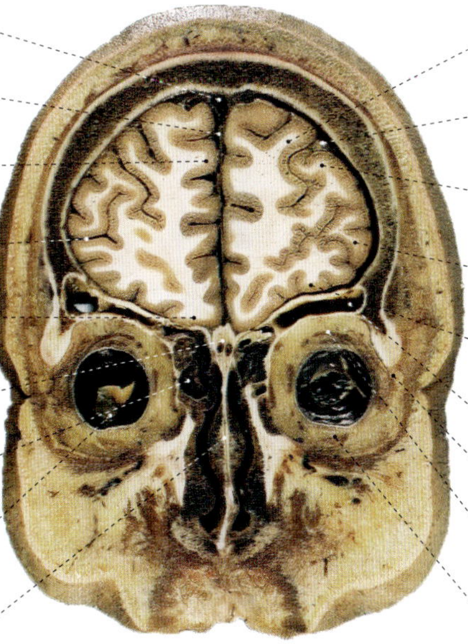

图 11-16　经额棘的冠状断面

Coronal section through frontal crest

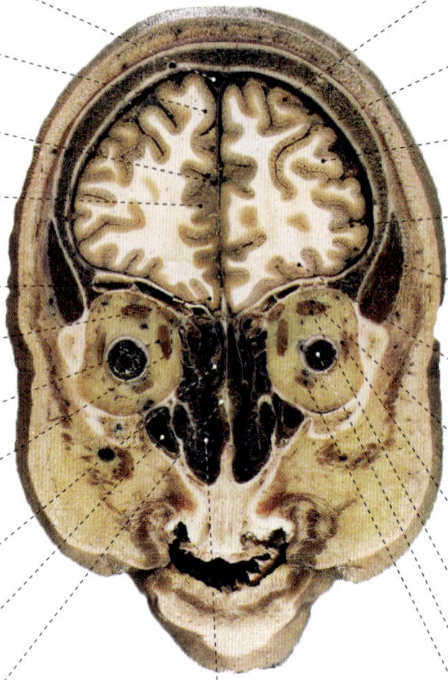

图 11–17　经鸡冠的冠状断面

Coronal section through crista galli

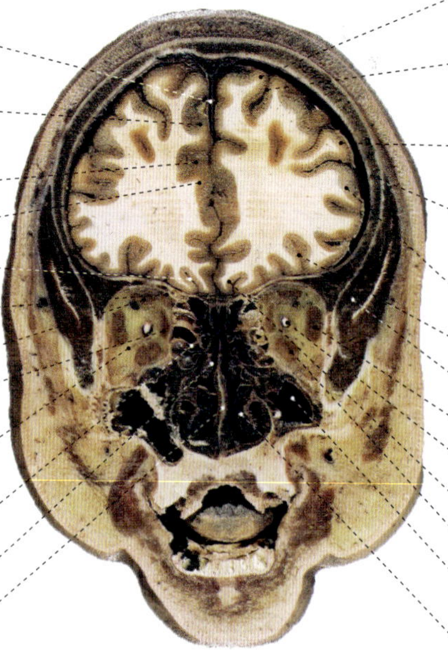

图 11–18　经上颌窦中份的冠状断面

Coronal section through middle part of maxillary sinus

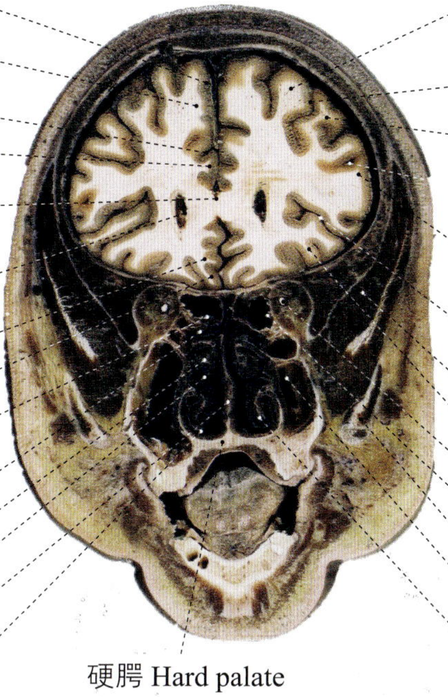

图 11–19　经胼胝体膝的冠状断面

Coronal section through genu of corpus callosum

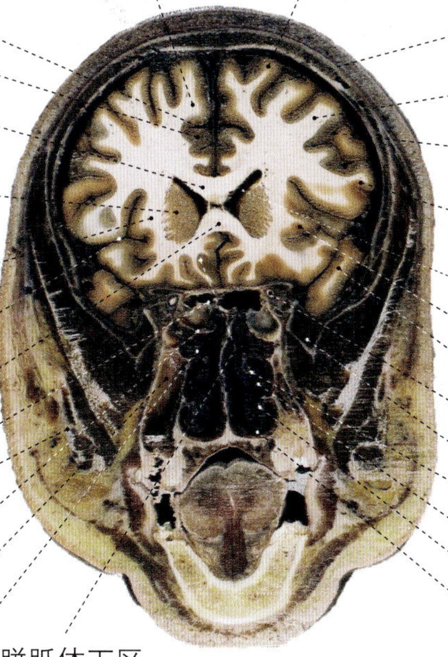

图 11–20　经颞极的冠状断面

Coronal section through temporal pole

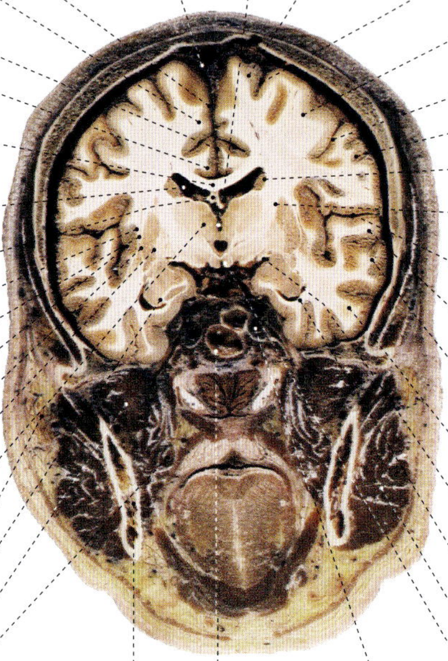

图 11–21　经乳头体的冠状断面

Coronal section through mamillary body

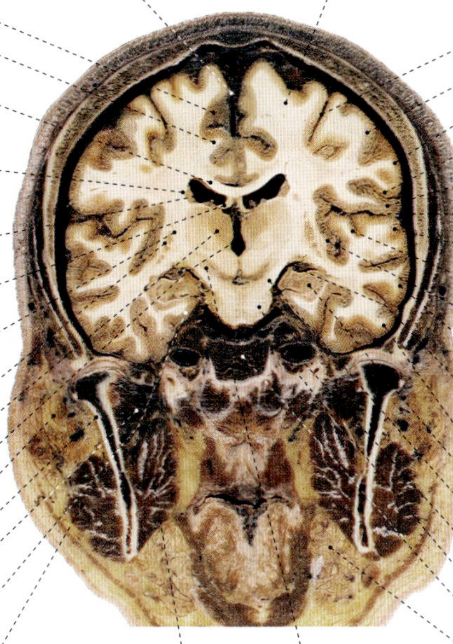

图 11–22 经红核和黑质的冠状断面

Coronal section through red nucleus and substantia nigra

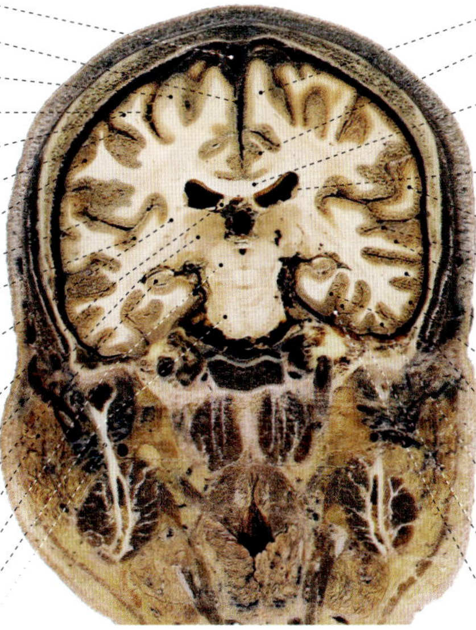

图 11–23 经脑桥的冠状断面

Coronal section through pons

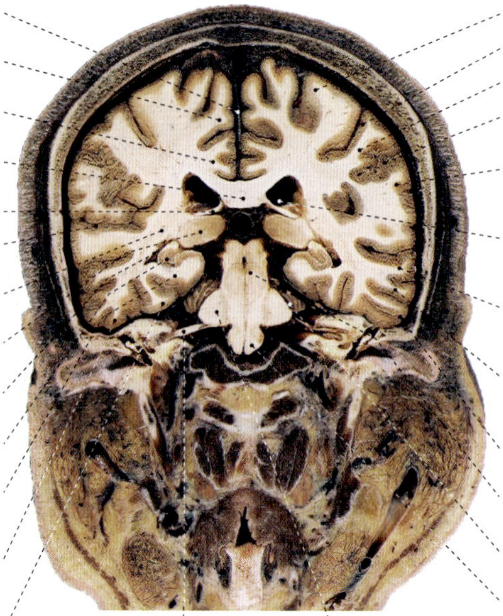

图 11–24　经小脑中脚的冠状断面

Coronal section through middle cerebellar peduncle

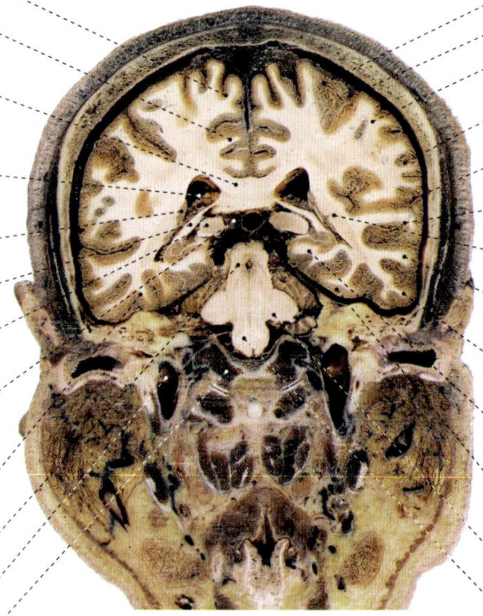

图 11–25　经颈静脉孔的冠状断面

Coronal section through jugular foramen

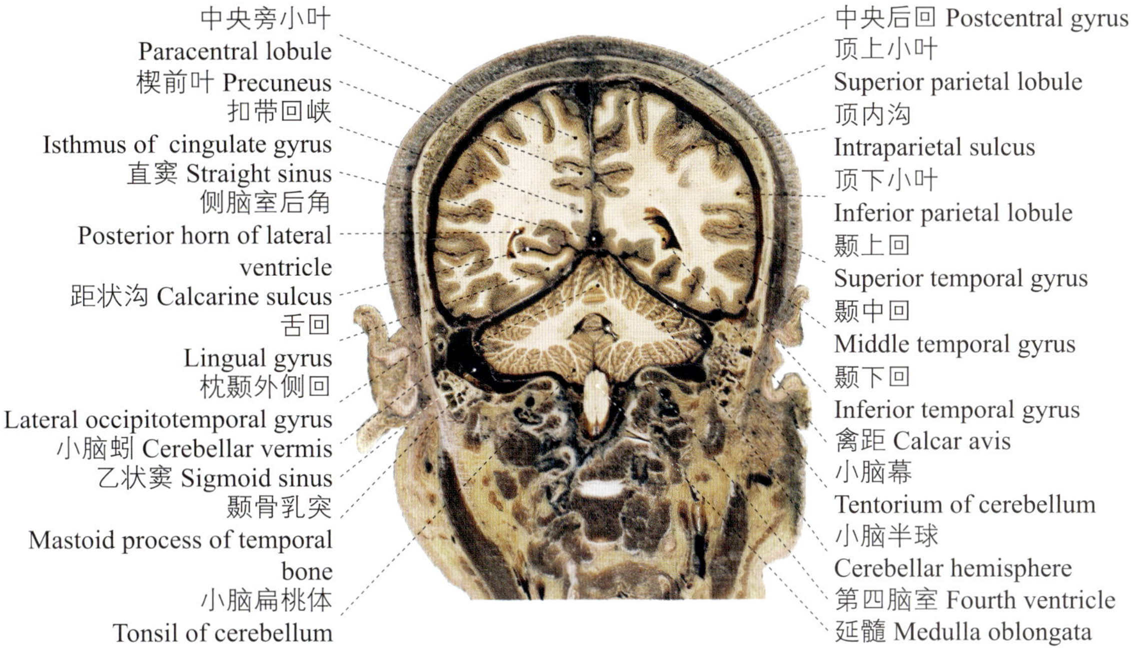

图 11–26　经侧脑室后角的冠状断面

Coronal section through posterior horn of lateral ventricle

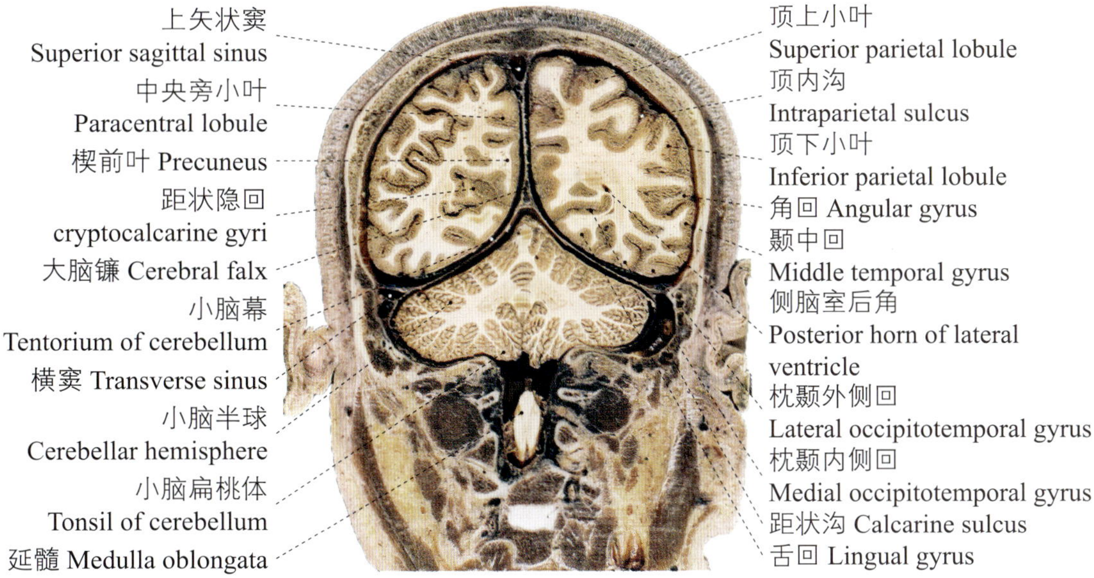

图 11–27　经距状隐回的冠状断面

Coronal section through cryptocalcarine gyri

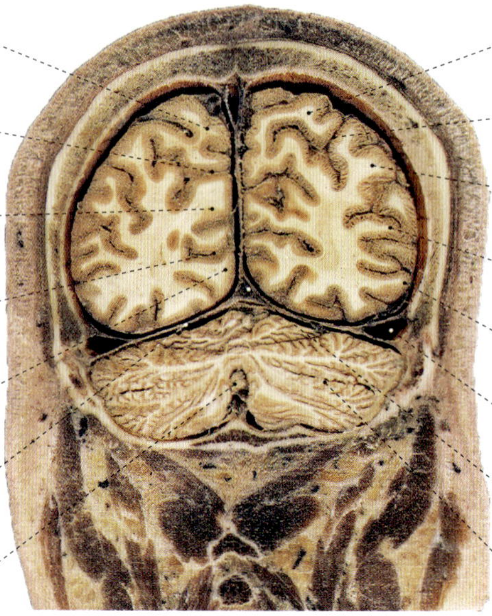

图 11–28　经直窦后份的冠状断面

Coronary section through posterior part of straight sinus

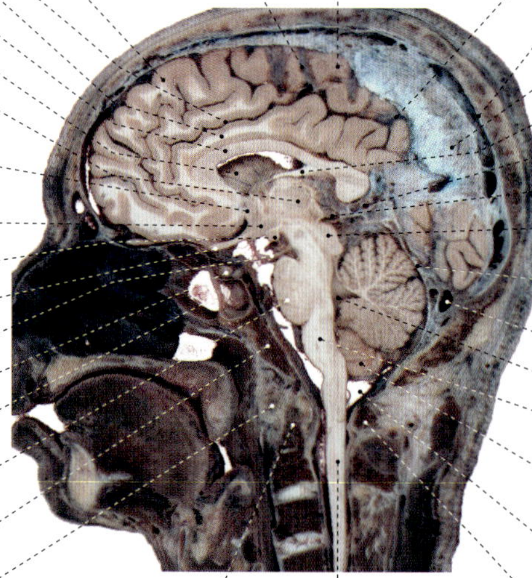

图 11–29　正中矢状面（左侧面观）

Median sagittal plane (Left lateral aspect)

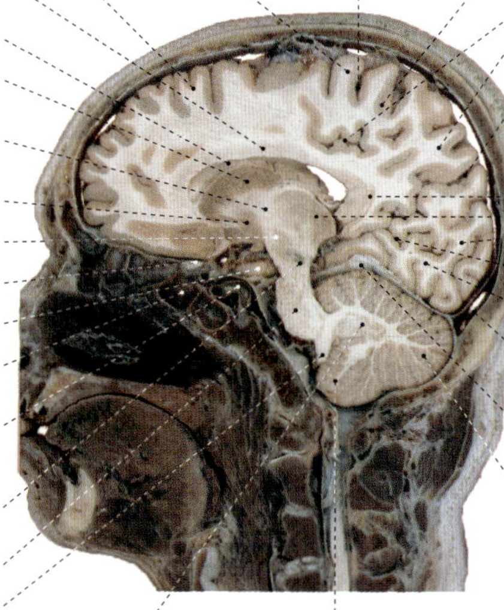

图 11-30　经右侧内囊膝的矢状断面

Sagittal section through right genu of internal capsule

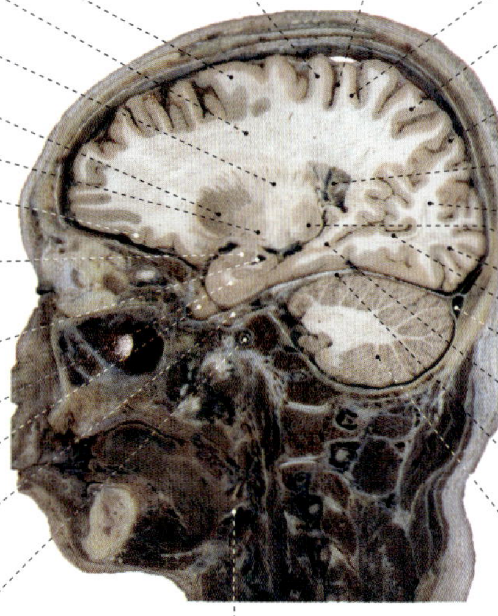

图 11-31　经右侧苍白球的矢状断面

Sagittal section through right globus pallidus

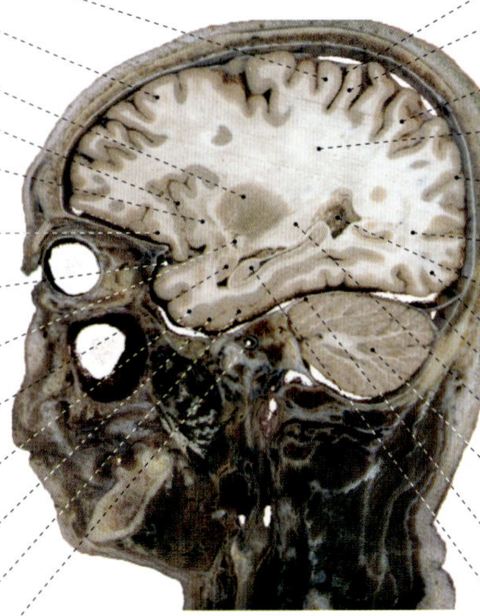

图 11–32　经右侧壳的矢状断面

Sagittal section through right putamen

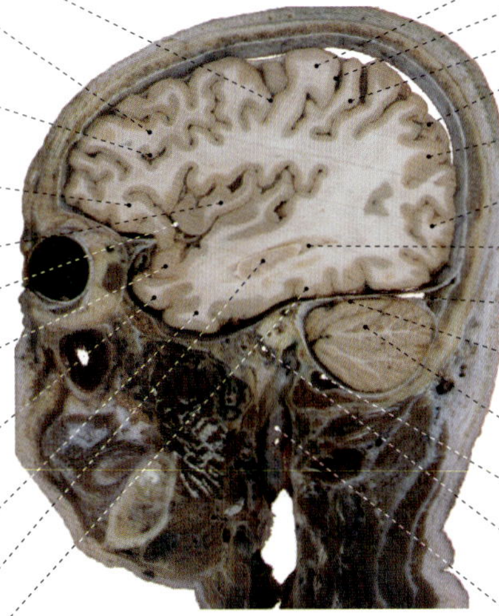

图 11–33　经右侧颈内静脉的矢状断面

Sagittal section through right internal jugular v.

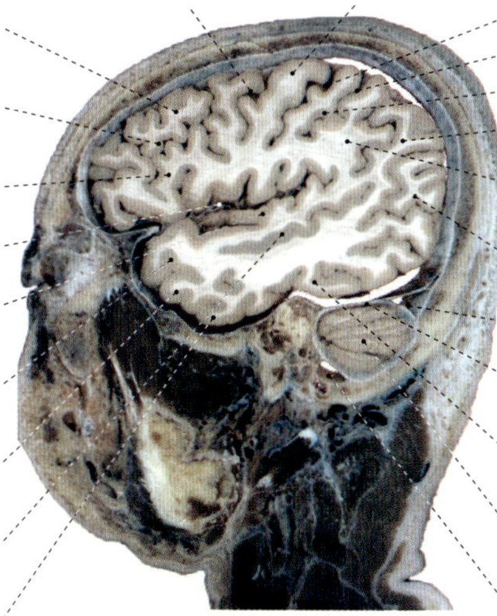

图 11–34　经右侧颞横回矢状断面

Sagittal section through right transverse temporal gyri

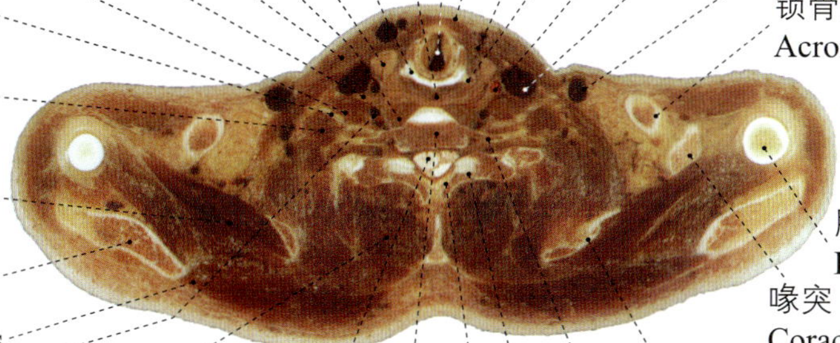

图 11–35　经环状软骨的横断面

Transverse section through cricoid cartilage

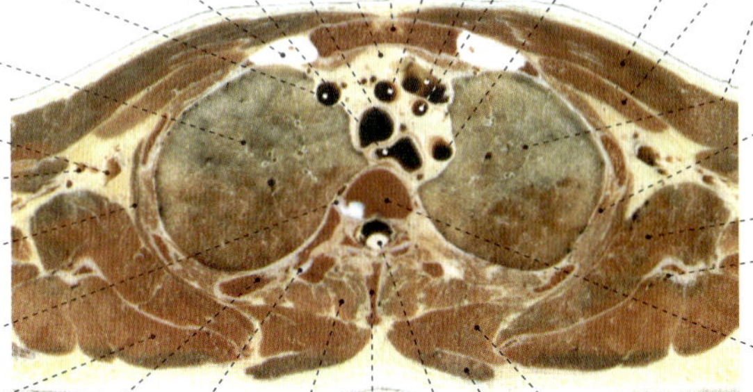

图 11–36　经第一肋软骨的横断面

Transverse section through first costal cartilage

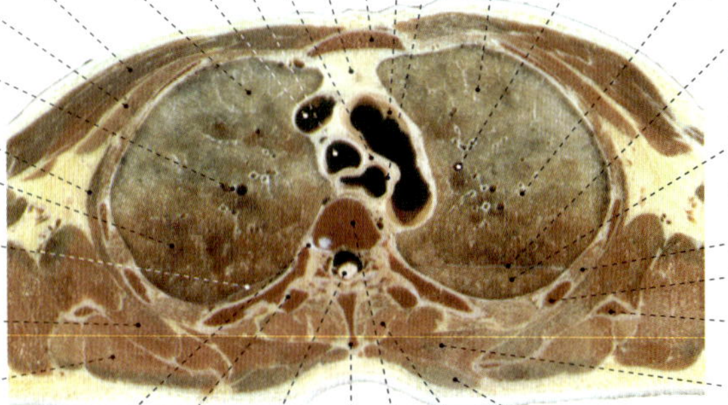

图 11–37　经主动脉弓的横断面

Transverse section through aortic arch

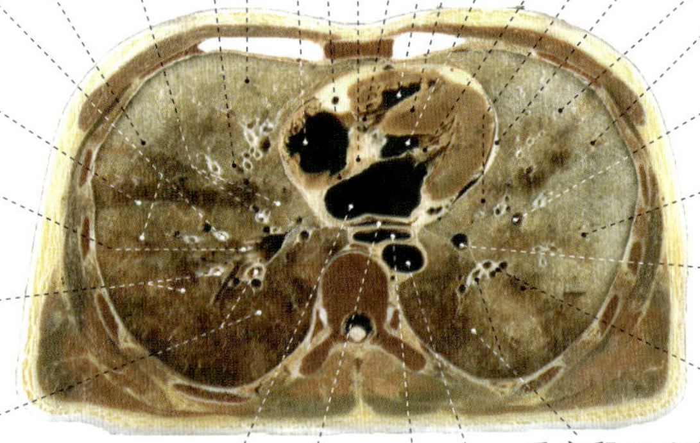

图 11–38　经卵圆窝的横断面

Transverse section through fossa ovalis

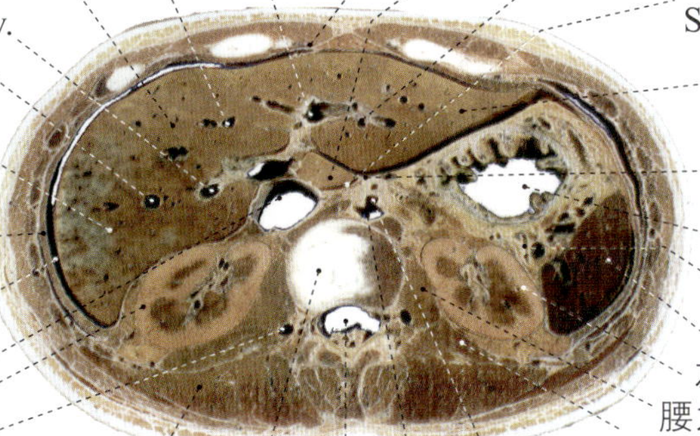

图 11–39　经腹腔干的横断面

Transverse section through celiac trunk

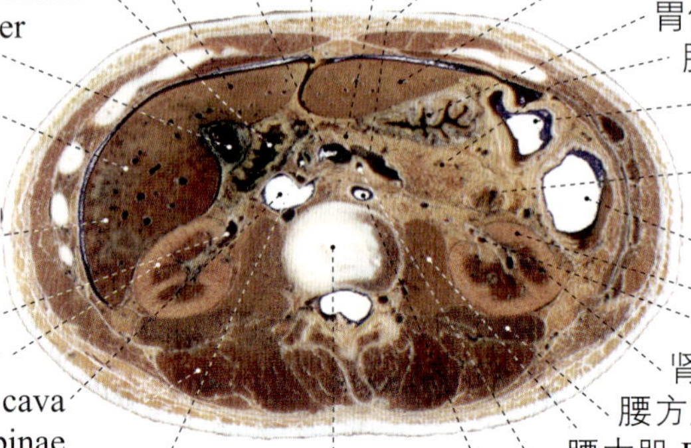

图 11–40　经肝门静脉合成处的横断面

Transverse section through synthesis site of hepatic portal v.

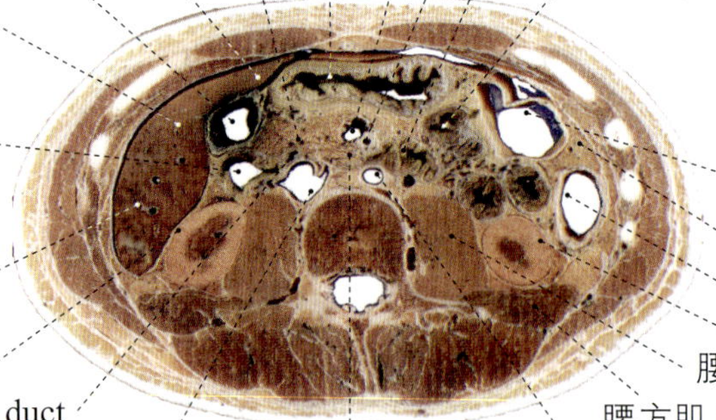

图 11–41　经第二腰椎体的横断面

Transverse section through body of second lumbar vertebra

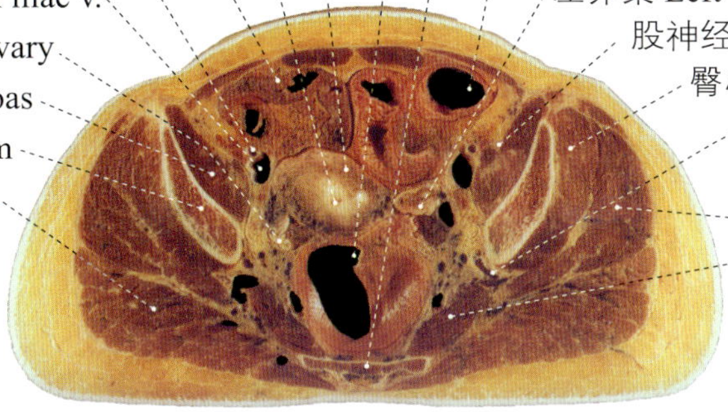

图 11–42　女性经坐骨大孔和子宫体的横断面

Female transverse section through greater sciatic foramen and uterine body

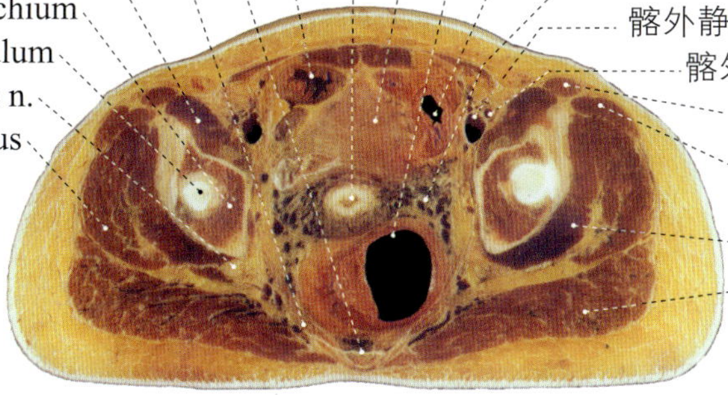

图 11–43　女性经尾骨和子宫颈的横断面

Female transverse section through coccyx and neck of uterus

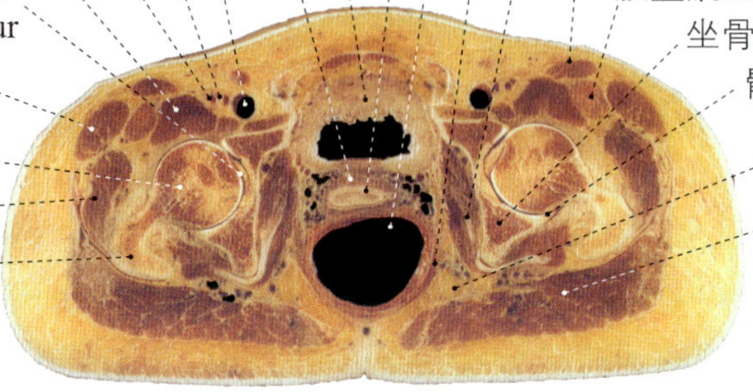

图 11–44　女性经股骨头的横断面

Female transverse section through femoral head

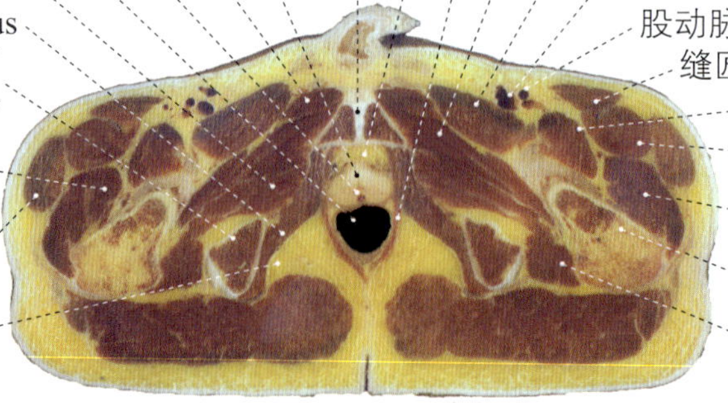

图 11–45　男性经耻骨联合下份的横断面

Male transverse section through lower part of Pubic symphysis

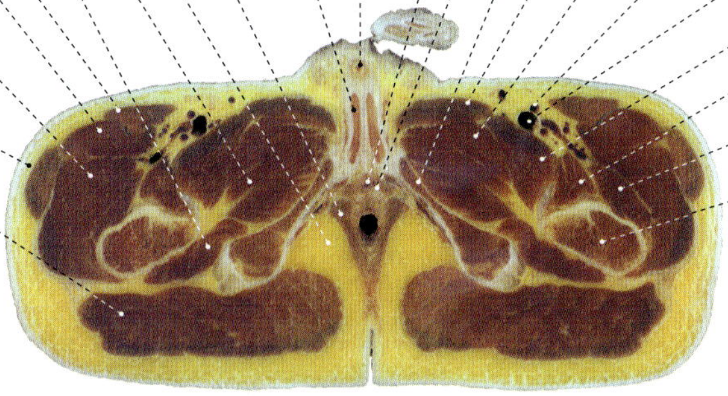

图 11–46 男性经坐骨支的横断面

Male transverse section through ramus of ischium

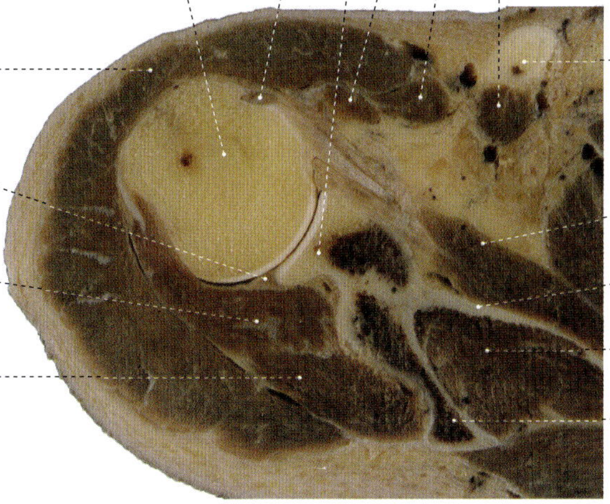

图 11–47 经肩胛冈的横断面

Transverse section through spine of scapula

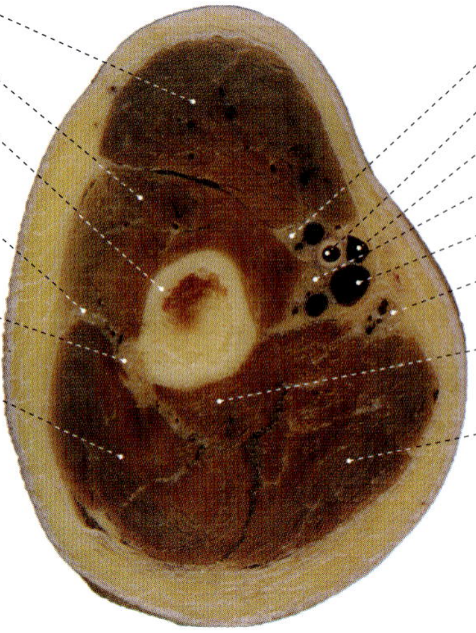

图 11–48　经臂中份的横断面

Transverse section through middle part of arm

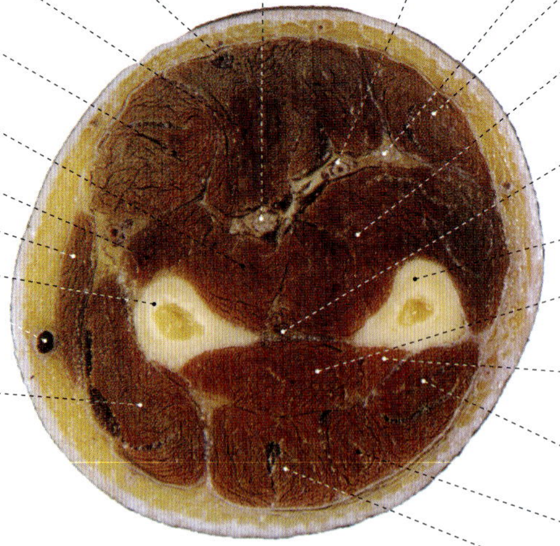

图 11–49　经前臂中份的横断面

Transverse section through middle part of forearm

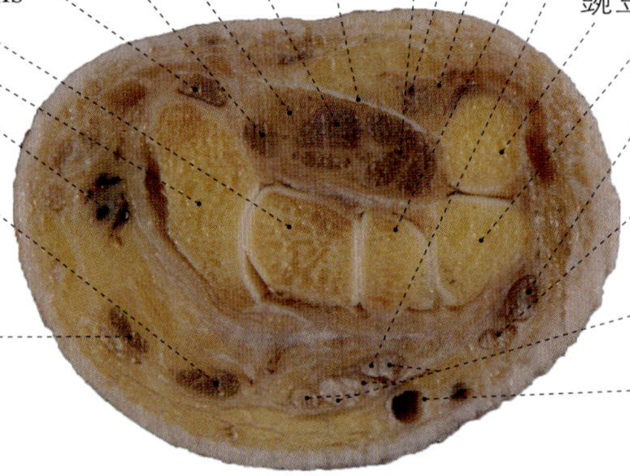

图 11–50　经腕管的横断面

Transverse section through carpal canal

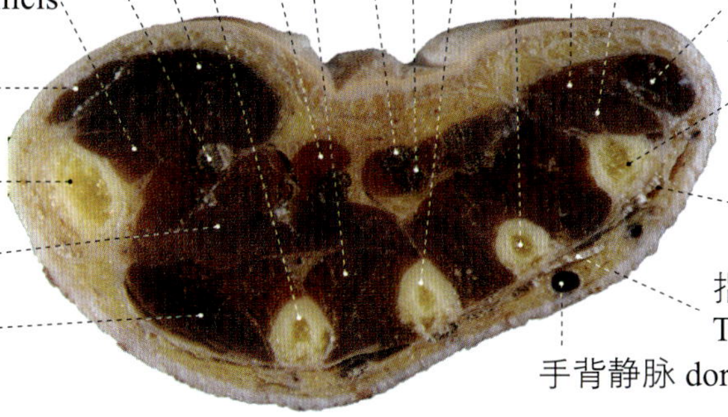

图 11–51　经掌骨中份的横断面

Transverse section through middle part of metacarpal bones

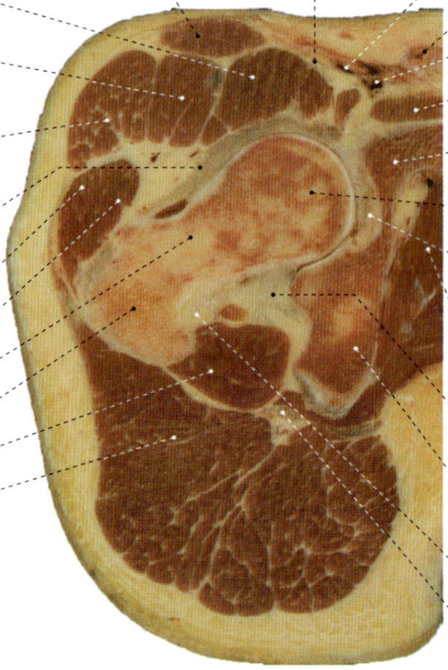

图 11–52　经髋关节的横断面

Transverse section through hip joint

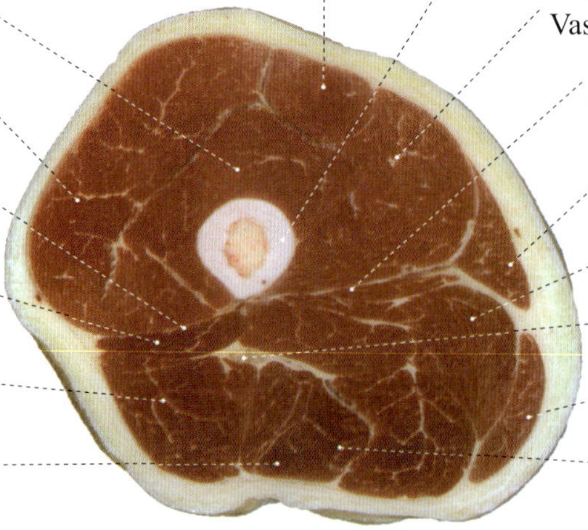

图 11–53　经股骨中份的横断面

Transverse section through middle part of femur